TELEMEDIC...

A NOVEL WAY TO FIGHT A

PANDEMIC

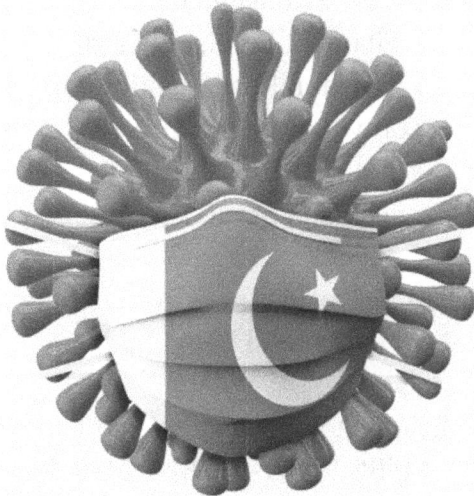

A SUCCESS STORY
FROM PAKISTAN

BY PROF W ANGUS WALLACE
& DR SUHAIL Y CHUGHTAI

Foreword by PROF JAY SAUNDERS MD

Founder: American Telemedicine Association

Professor of Medicine: John Hopkins School of Medicine, USA

Filament
Publishing

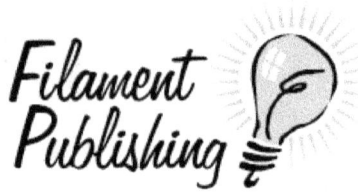

Published by
Filament Publishing Ltd
16, Croydon Road, Beddington,
Croydon, Surrey CR0 4PA
+44(0) 20 8688 2598
www.filamentpublishing.com

Telemedicine - A novel way to fight a pandemic
ISBN 978-1-913623-21-0

Printed in the UK by 4Edge

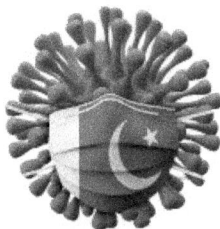

An unprecedented problem
A novel solution

The Covid 19 pandemic took the world by surprise. Even those advanced countries with a well-established healthcare infrastructure were caught out by the speed that the virus spread and took hold.

As a new virus, very little was known about its properties, how it was spread, and the short and long-term effects on health. The death toll was growing fast. The world needed answers, and fast. What was clear from the beginning was that existing healthcare structures were not adequate to manage the situation. Every country reacted in different ways.

In Pakistan, The Punjab Government deployed "Smart Lockdown" as a policy to limit the Corona epidemic in March 2020. The essential services of the Patient-Doctor physical visit posed the risk of spreading the Corona epidemic. However, in addition to the growing numbers was a real danger that people rushing to the medical facilities (Hospital and Family Doctors) to obtain advice for suspected Corona virus symptoms, could have flooded the Government hospitals and private clinics.

No matter what the crisis, in the moment of most need a solution presented itself.

This is the story of what happened.

Table of Contents

Foreword
Prof Dr Jay Saunders
M.D., FACP, FACAA&I, FATA

*Founder & President Emeritus:
American Telemedicine Association.
Professor of Medicine (Adj): Johns
Hopkins School of Medicine Former
Director of Telemedicine: Medical
College of Georgia, USA   CEO: The
Global Telemedicine Group, USA*

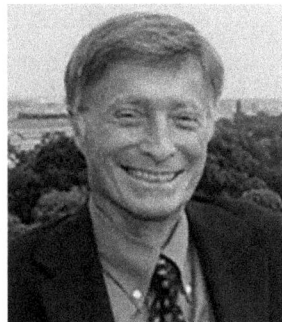

It gives me great pleasure to pen a few lines about the subject of the book, "Telemedicine, a Novel way to Fight a Pandemic", authored by Prof Angus Wallace and Dr Suhail Chughtai, both orthopaedic surgeons based in the UK. Although Telemedicine has existed for many years, the COVID-19 pandemic has significantly accelerated the pace of adoption. I am aware of the success story that emerged from Pakistan where the deployment of the "Telemedicine 24/7 Helpline" managed to prevent the crowding of hospitals and thus reduce the spread of the virus. I am sure that this was a contributing factor in Pakistan getting included as one of the seven most successful nations in controlling the spread of this virus in the first wave of the pandemic.

Dr Suhail Chughtai, the Founding Chairman of Medical City Online, responded to the COVID-19 crisis in Pakistan and helped the country of his origin by converting one of his Telemedicine software products to an Instant Connect Corona Telemedicine Helpline, published as a website named www.Doctors247.online.

Additionally, Dr Chughtai led the software training network from London for over 350 doctors. His team in Pakistan helped set up a chain of regional Telemedicine Hubs housed within campuses of various Medical Universities keeping the central control centre at the University of Health Sciences, Lahore, Pakistan which was visited by the President of Pakistan a few weeks after the inauguration for a formal project briefing.

The idea worked as planned since young doctors who were brought into the framework not only learned how to use the software quickly but managed to provide free medical advice to over 530,000 people. The Helpline's success supported the lockdown measures taken by the Government of Pakistan to limit the spread of the pandemic which otherwise would have been a national disaster in the face of a limited supply of ventilators in a country of 220 million people.

I congratulate both authors of the book "Telemedicine, a Novel to Fight a Pandemic" for their initiative showing how Telemedicine can be used in other parts of the world where medical expertise in dealing with a crisis might be limited.

In my personal view, Telemedicine should be viewed as an additional resource in the day-to-day practice of medicine, and of particular importance when time, distance, availability and convenience are factors in limiting a patient's access to the healthcare delivery system.

PROLOGUE

Chaudhary Muhammad Sarwar
immediate past Governor of Punjab

Mr Nafees Zakaria
immediate past High Commissioner
of Pakistan to the UK

Mr Charles Lowe
Past President Telemedicine
Department, The Royal Society of
Medicine, London, UK

Chaudhary Muhammad Sarwar
immediate past Governor of Punjab, Pakistan

It gives me pleasure to write the prologue of this book authored by Prof Dr Angus Wallace and Dr Suhail Chughtai. Right from its inception, I have been strongly associated with the project of setting up the Telemedicine 24/7 Helpline Centres in Pakistan when it was needed most at the vulnerable period of the COVID-19 pandemic reaching the country in the first quarter of 2020.

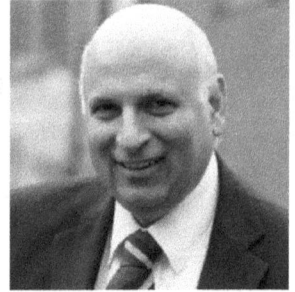

The very idea of using Telemedicine to limit the spread of the pandemic was put to action in a very methodical way. I personally supported and pro-actively became involved in implementing the Telemedicine helpline centres in Punjab, which is the largest and most heavily populated province of Pakistan. Teaching Hospitals, attached to medical colleges, were particularly involved, in line with the policy of the Prime Minister Imran Khan whose main objective was to limit people's movement between home and hospitals during the lock down.

I am glad to express that all the medical universities responded to my call fervently in support of the Telemedicine Helpline project to facilitate local Telemedicine Hubs at their respective campuses. We also setup Telemedicine specifically for Women, The Pink Telemedicine centre and one to deal solely with Mental Health issues.

Dr Khurram Shahzad and Dr Humayun Taimur along with my team at the Governor house including Miss Rabia

Zia and Chaudhary Ansar Farooq facilitated every logistic requirement such as the installation of hardware, setting up training facilities of doctors on software and parallel logistic support for the service providers.

Dr Suhail Chughtai customised his Telemedicine Software, re-designing it in 3 days to a Telemedicine Helpline with in-built Corona Scoring where a doctor could categorise a patient during the Teleconsultation. The simplicity of design of his Telemedicine website, www.Doctors247.online minimised the learning curve for both doctors and patients with quick adaptation to a relatively new method of patient-doctor visit in Pakistan.

It was encouraging to see the results of the effort with Pakistan emerging as one of the seven most successful countries in the world to have fought the pandemic efficiently. I believe that the timely inclusion of the Telemedicine 24/7 Helpline contributed to Prime Minister Imran Khan's policy in controlling the pandemic in our country.

It is pertinent to note that nearly 10,000 doctors, consultants, paramedic staff, and final year MBBS students volunteered themselves for the Telemedicine 24/7 Helpline working in shifts and without any financial benefit. More than half a million people benefited from the Telemedicine 24/7 Helpline project which was inaugurated by me at the University of Health Sciences under the supervision of VC Prof Dr Javed Akram on 18th March 2020.

The whole team involved in setting up this Telemedicine helpline deserves special appreciation as their timely effort and coordinated action, I believe, saved Pakistan a large number of lives.

Mr Nafees Zakaria

Immediate past High Commissioner of Pakistan to the UK

In my capacity as the High Commissioner for Pakistan, I am privileged and take great pride in contributing my comments to the informative book, "Telemedicine - A Novel Way to Fight a Pandemic" authored by Prof Dr Angus Wallace, an esteemed UK Professor and Dr Suhail Chughtai, a distinguished and accomplished doctor of Pakistani heritage, both Orthopaedic Surgeons based in the UK.

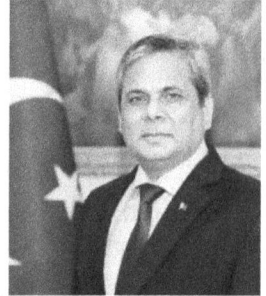

Revolution in digital technology in the past four decades has transformed the world in a manner that no other field of science and technology has ever done. The vast universe has shrunk to be dubbed as a "global village". Access to every piece of information and virtual contacts on the internet has become just a matter of a 'click'.

Telemedicine is one of the most useful outcomes of the evolution of digital healthcare technology. It gives me great pleasure to recall the days ten years ago when Dr Chughtai and I discussed the idea of Telemedicine to reach out to the less privileged people in Pakistan, who faced difficulty in accessing the medical facilities for a variety of reason, not specific to Pakistan only. The field was wide open for Dr Chughtai to explore and exploit to the beneficiary (i.e. the common man/woman)'s advantage.

Awareness and institutionalisation of Dr Chughtai's Telemedicine initiative by way of an understanding with the

Punjab Government has benefited over half a million people in Pakistan. The ten-year journey of Telemedicine through Dr Chughtai's promotional efforts proved its real worth and efficacy when the pandemic COVID-19 struck the world.

Pakistan, a country of 220 million people, was lauded by the WHO Chief for not only suppressing COVID-19 but also keeping the economy afloat. In Pakistan's COVID-19 related achievement, Telemedicine played a significant role. Apparently, COVID-19 does not seem to be disappearing in the foreseeable future. Therefore, dependence on Telemedicine is bound to grow for obvious reasons.

Telemedicine together with Telediagnosis and with the effective use of emerging technology, Artificial Intelligence (AI), will inevitably revolutionise the field of medical science in the times ahead. Telemedicine, Telediagnosis and Teleclinics may become a "neo-normal" in the near future.

I thank Dr Suhail Chughtai for allowing me the opportunity to add my thoughts. I congratulate both of the worthy authors for their accomplishment in the field of Telehealth.

Mr CHARLES LOWE MBA

Past President of the Royal Society of Medicine UK's Telemedicine & eHealth Section. CEO Digital Health & Care Alliance, Chair of the Board of Trustees, Citizens Online, Business Development Advisor of Medical City Online, UK.

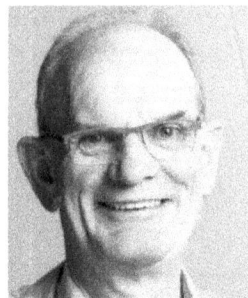

Charles has a background in digital health, working in both public & private sectors. His recent work has centred on the regulation & assessment of mHealth apps. He is also a Contributing Editor to www.telecareaware.com, a Special Adviser to both NICE and the CQC, and he is the organiser of the London Health Technology Forum. He consults for Humetrix Inc on app-related matters. He chairs Citizens Online, the digital inclusion charity.

Significant care pathway improvements in medicine that disrupt organisational structures and change doctor-patient relationships typically require a crisis of some sort to become embedded.

Telemedicine was no exception. COVID-19 has provided the impetus for that change, from which there will be little going back because the benefits to patients and clinicians are so great.

For patients, time saved travelling and waiting, being seen much quicker, and in accessing expert opinion are all hugely attractive. The benefits to clinicians are equally good, with many now able to consult from home.

As also the Chair of an organisation, "Citizens Online" with a strong focus on inclusion, the unexpected benefit that appeals to me most is that clinicians no longer have to wear masks when consulted online, so those who rely on lip-reading are no longer excluded.

This book, "Telemedicine, A Novel Way to Fight a Pandemic", authored by Prof Angus Wallace and Dr Suhail Chughtai, describes the benefits of Virtual healthcare in great detail during situations of a spreading community infection, resulting from the recent COVID 19 pandemic.

Epilogue

World Congress of Overseas Pakistanis UK

Association of Pakistani Physicians & Surgeons UK

Akhuwat Pakistan

Jump Start Pakistan

Medical City Online UK

Allama Iqbal Medical College Alumni UK

World Congress of Overseas Pakistanis - UK

Immediate past Chairperson: Mr Qamar Raza Syed
Executive Director: Mr Arif Anis Malik

I came across the intriguing manuscript "Telemedicine, a Novel way to Fight a Pandemic", authored by Prof Dr Angus Wallace and Dr Suhail Chughtai, orthopaedic surgeons based in the UK. I think this book is one of the most thought-provoking works on this emerging discipline.

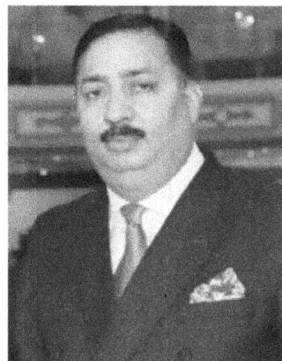

Telemedicine, a phenomenon defined by the authors as "rapid access to shared and remote medical expertise by ICT (Information Communication Technology), no matter where the patient or relevant information is located". The authors regard Telemedicine as a part of health telematics. This demonstrates a technology-driven definition of the term Telemedicine, so the focus of the book itself is similarly technological in nature. However, what makes it unique is its application in the recent coronavirus pandemic.

A significant issue in ICT systems, and especially for ICT in health and medicine, is supporting communication between various partners. Delivering integrated healthcare is an area where enhanced, efficient, and cost-effective communication between professionals, and between professionals and patients, plays a very important role. However, in medicine, the ease of use of telecommunication systems, of information sources, of feedback, and integration of services is after many years of work, still not sufficiently well developed. Thus, books in this area are needed at this time.

Pakistan emerged less affected than other countries from the corona virus pandemic. Even the Imperial College London projected a horrific picture, but by the end of September 2020, the cases are much less than expected with a low mortality ratio. Dr Chughtai, who has been rightly conferred the Foreign Minister Honours in August 2020, and his team, contributed vigorously through Telemedicine and hundreds, and thousands of people in Pakistan have benefited.

This book is an excellent addition to the application of this emerging discipline and sets it as a success story that can inspire this revolution globally. On behalf of the World Congress of Overseas Pakistani, I congratulate both authors on this wonderful contribution to Digital Health.

Association of Pakistani Physicians & Surgeons, UK

President: Mr Shakeel Puri
Immediate past Chairperson: Dr Shaheena Anjum

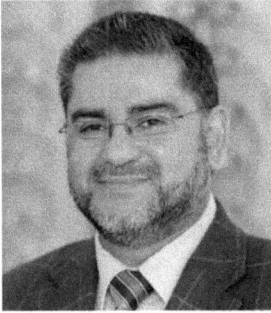

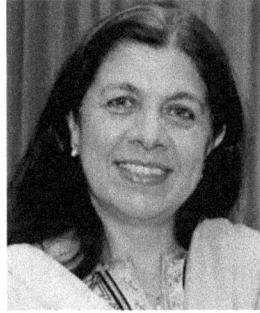

The COVID-19 pandemic has changed the world as we understood it. The pandemic impacted human life in all its aspects around the globe. If one says that there was a pre-COVID-19 world and there will be a post-COVID-19 world, one would be not far off from the truth. The COVID-19 pandemic started as a global health crisis; it slowly engulfed the global economy and now is dictating mankind to reassess the way it has evolved and learnt how to live.

The impact of COVID-19 cannot be felt more strongly anywhere else than in health care services. It has pushed the health care delivery model into uncharted territory. The existing models of health care service delivery have been exposed in a somewhat unexpected manner. The changes, which would have taken decades to come, have been fast-forwarded. Innovative use of the available technologies, especially information technology, has come to the forefront, providing us with new opportunities to rethink our strategy and methodology for the future delivery of our health care service.

One such 'fast-forwarded' the use of technology in providing health care services since the COVID-19 pandemic is Telemedicine. Prof Angus Wallace and Dr Suhail Chughtai have done a wonderful job by publishing their work of combing the experience and expertise from two different health care systems during this COVID-19 crisis using the medium of Telemedicine.

"Telemedicine: A success story from Pakistan" is indeed a ground-breaking work as far as the future of health care service delivery in Pakistan is concerned and we are proud to see Dr Suhail Chughtai design this Telemedicine Helpline project as he is also the Director of Digital Health & Telemedicine Sector of our organization (APPSUK).

We, on behalf of APPS UK Board of Directors, congratulate the authors and their team for such an excellent job which, I am sure, will go a long way in further improving health care services in Pakistan in the times to come.

AKHUWAT, PAKISTAN

Founder and Executive Director: Dr Amjad Saqib

I am delighted to appreciate Prof Angus Wallace and Dr Suhail Chughtai, who have taken the initiative to author this book, "A Novel Way to Fight a Pandemic". I am aware of the project's need and its methodical deployment right from its start on 18th March 2020 at the University of Health Sciences, Lahore Pakistan, where I participated in the inauguration ceremony. The event was also attended by the Honourable Chaudhry Mohammad Sarwar, past Governor Punjab, who has taken a keen interest in the promotion of the project subsequently.

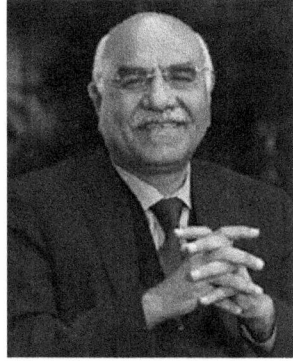

The Telemedicine 24/7 Helpline providing crucial support to Punjab's response to COVID-19 was a necessary and timely intervention. Dr Suhail Chughtai was able to devise a support system that encouraged people to stay at home and still have a medical opinion if they were showing any symptoms of the virus. Considering our inadequate resources, it would have been catastrophic if we had allowed the virus to spread like it did in other countries of the region.

The innovative and apt use of the Telemedicine service to limit the spread of the pandemic was received well by medical universities in the province which helped Dr Suhail Chughtai and his team to set up a chain of Telemedicine Hubs while training doctors to enable them in providing efficient and round the clock free medical advice.

The simple interface of the website (www.Doctors247. online) enhanced it's usability, thus supporting hundreds of people in the most testing times. These poor people also included beneficiaries of Akhuwat, the largest interest-free micro-finance program in the world.

I congratulate both Dr Suhail Chughtai and Prof Angus Wallace on their efforts to support Pakistan's people in reducing the rate of the instance of COVID-19. This book will serve to preserve the Telemedicine COVID 24/7 Helpline as a practical example for future policymakers and healthcare professionals in designing innovative approaches to solving other complex issues in the health sector.

JUMP START PAKISTAN

Chairman: Mr Amjad Pervez

As Chairman of Jump Start Pakistan, I am delighted indeed and honoured to write in support of Prof Dr Angus Wallace and Dr Suhail Chughtai who have taken the much-needed effort to author this wonderfully informative book, "A Novel Way to Fight a Pandemic". I recognise the project's scope and its role for the well-being of the Pakistani public at large. The methodical deployment right from its launch on 18th March 2020 at the University of Health Sciences, Lahore Pakistan and its further take-off is a success story from day one and onwards.

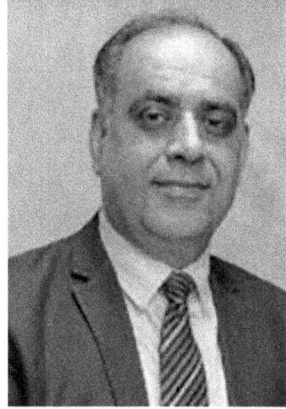

This Telemedicine 24/7 Helpline to fight Corona Pandemic was an appropriate and timely modern technology-driven response by Dr Suhail Chughtai, Chairman of Medical City Online, who sensed the pulse of the moment. Considering the lack of ventilators for the given population size, it would have been unmanageable if COVID-19 had spread as wide as it did in neighbouring countries where the death toll was sadly phenomenally higher.

The sensible and innovative use of Telemedicine service to limit the spread of the pandemic was responded to well by the medical universities in the province which helped Dr Suhail Chughtai and his team on the ground to set up a chain of Telemedicine Hubs.

It is known to me that the Doctors were trained on this Doctors 24/7 Online software to provide an efficient, round the clock free medical advice to people during the first phase of the Corona Pandemic Lockdown. Doctors and patients took up the service with ease enabling a significant success of this project's website www.Doctors247.online.

My heartfelt congratulations to Dr Suhail Chughtai and Prof Angus Wallace on putting the experience of this valuable project in the form of a book, leaving an example project of Healthcare Technology that saved lives in large numbers.

Also, it will record to demonstrate that there are still good people in this world who use their knowledge, skills and expertise for the betterment of humanity rather than self-interest.

MEDICAL CITY ONLINE UK

CEO: Mr Bud Zborowski   MBA

Bud Zborowski is CEO and Advisor for Medical City Online. His executive business career spans more than three decades and is well-grounded in healthcare operations with expertise leading business growth strategy built around emerging medical technologies and innovative healthcare business solutions.

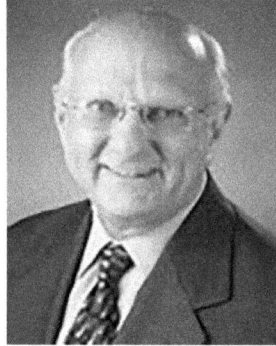

He is the former global market director for Telemedicine at Polycom, Inc., a $1 billion international voice-video-data technology leader. He served on a number of industry boards including the American Telemedicine Association and participated as an invited Charter Member at the Washington D.C. based Centre for Health Transformation.

Before the COVID-19 pandemic, people were getting accustomed to using online video to communicate with business, family, and friends via Skype, Zoom and the like.

In March 2020 with little advanced warning the mobile devices took on an expanded role in everyone's lives and the "Corona Telemedicine Helpline" setup on Doctors 24/7 Online website, backed up by telephone lines became a household name. In the background is a powerful story about how public health made history, leveraging the ubiquitous mobile device, Telemedicine, and the patient-doctor relationship to deliver lifesaving advice and medical care.

The Opportunity: By its nature, Telemedicine has been practicing long-distance "social distancing" for almost three decades delivering care to outreach areas in Canada and Alaska as well as in rural US populations. So, when pandemic-grade personal distancing and lockdowns surfaced overnight, virtual care quickly became the perfect vehicle for pandemic-era public health communications and medical care. In Pakistan, this translated into establishing a state wide Telemedicine-based COVID-19 Hotline designed to serve the city and rural populations in Pakistan alike. It was a fresh, bold, and ground-breaking initiative.

The Challenge: As with all innovation, implementation challenges surface. In this case, three stood out. First, implementation had to be immediate; saving time meant saving lives. Second, it needed 100% buy-in from large major stakeholders: Government, Medical academics, Physicians and Private enterprise. Third, success demanded an at-the-ready, best-in-class, clinically tested Telemedicine software that was easy to use, scalable and drove results. Enter Medical City Online UK Telemedicine software group and Pakistani based Citrus Telemedicine, a healthcare delivery project via Telemedicine, led by Dr Suhail Chughtai who is an Orthopaedic Surgeon and Telehealth Expert, based in the UK.

The Future: This particular public health project held an important key and go-to-market advantage. All stakeholders shared a common sense of urgency and the vision to raise health standards for the country. Within weeks a functioning public health initiative was born, implemented, and began handling tens of thousands citizen COVID-19 inquiries all conducted within the protection bubble of accepted social distancing and medical confidentiality.

The experience also provides us with a view into the future of medical care delivery for Pakistan. The long-term success of this project has the opportunity to set the bar for incorporating what is considered the "next normal" in global healthcare.

I congratulate both Prof Angus Wallace and Dr Suhail Chughtai for the effort in capturing this innovative project into a book, a story that has a lesson for the countries where COVID-19 caused significant loss of human life.

LLAMA IQBAL MEDICAL COLLEGE ALUMNI UK

Dr Usman Khan
Consultant General Surgeon UK,
Chairman Allama Iqbal Medical College Alumni UK

Dr Ayaz Asghar
Ophthalmologist UK, Ex Chair & Director
Allama Iqbal Medical College Alumni UK

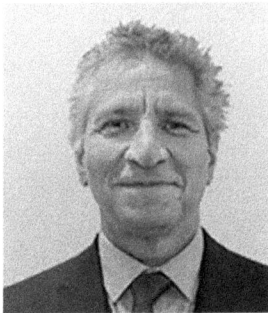

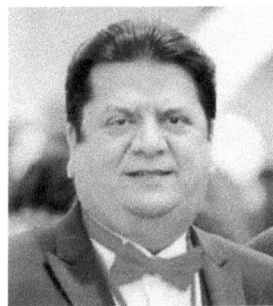

It is a pleasure to write a few lines for one of the two authors, Prof Angus Wallace & Dr Suhail Chughtai for the book, "Telemedicine, a novel way to fight pandemic".

We have known Suhail for over 30 years from his medical college days. He has made tremendous progress over the years because of his innovative mind, hard work and resilience. Very early in his career, Suhail realised the importance of digital technology and diverted all his energies to this cause.

Suhail has created several digital healthcare projects including establishing the "Telemedicine Corona 24/7 Helpline during Lockdown in Pakistan" which helped enormously to mitigate risks of Corona pandemic spread in Pakistan while reducing the crowding in the hospital out-patient departments.

Suhail has been working in conjunction with the Government of Punjab province to provide free online consultations from doctors abroad during the coronavirus pandemic. This helped save thousands of lives and has also educated young and old in Pakistan.

We, at Allama Iqbal Medical College Alumni, are very proud of Suhail's achievements and his contribution to the COVID-19 Pandemic limitation in Pakistan through his innovative idea of Telemedicine based 24/7 Helpline service.

www.AIMCAUK.org

Tribute to the Fallen Hero in the fight against COVID

Late Prof Dr Mustafa Kamal Pasha

Vice-Chancellor, Nishtar Medical University (NMU), Multan
Professor of Surgery, Incharge of Corona Telemedicine
Hub at NMU

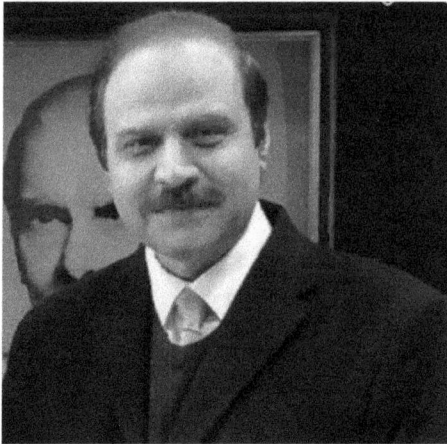

Obituary by Dr Suhail Chughtai

COVID-19 Pandemic took the lives of a significant number of medical professionals who put their lives at risk and kept serving their duties as the frontline healthcare force. Prof Mustafa Kamal Pasha was one such hero whom we lost at the hands of this pandemic.

Prof Mustapha Pasha was the son of Prof Dr Muhammad Kamal, Professor of Cardiology who also served as a Principal of Nishtar Medical College Multan. He completed his FRCS from Ireland and returned to Nishtar Medical College in 1993 to serve Pakistan with his excellent academic and clinical skills.

He was appointed as the first Vice-Chancellor of Nishtar Medical University Multan, a position he was still serving till he breathed last.

Prof Mustapha Pasha stood as a symbol of motivation for the medical students, post-graduate students and colleagues alike. With his captivating smile, dedicated support, and humble attitude, he exemplified true leadership qualities.

Prof Mustafa Kamal Pasha lost his fight against COVID-19 on 15th July, 2020. He took voluntary home self-isolation after the appearance of early symptoms around four weeks before his demise though later shifted to a private hospital in Multan upon developing slight breathing difficulties. As his condition deteriorated, Prof Pasha was later shifted to Lahore at a highly specialized ICU. Sadly, his lungs kept deteriorating, and on 6th July, the team of doctors decided to place Dr Pasha on extracorporeal membrane oxygenation (ECMO). Prof Pasha sadly expired nine days later after fighting with the deadly condition.

Prof Mustapha Kamal Pasha, with his captivating smile, carried a reputation of motivating people around him. He exemplified leadership skills and raised standard of education at the Nishtar Medical University. During the process of setting up the Telemedicine hub at his institution, a day before the inauguration, I spoke to him on the phone from the UK where his voice was full of enthusiasm and positive energy, and he ensured to provide all the best resources for the Telemedicine Hub for the Doctors 24/7 Helpline at his university computer lab.

His response to our call for a local Telemedicine Hub was assertive yet enriched with humility and kindness left an impression on me before we closed the call.

During his illness, he kept his morale up as is evident in the video recorded on 22nd July in a private hospital in Multan where he said with his well-known energetic smile, "I am fine, having tea and will be back soon".

Prof Mustapha Kamal Pasha's services were remembered for his dedication in the fight against COVID-19 while putting his life at risk in the line of duty through several nominations of high civil awards by the Government of Pakistan.

We shall remember you Prof Mustapha Kamal Pasha for all you did for the medical profession and your patients. May your soul stay blessed and rest in peace. Amen.

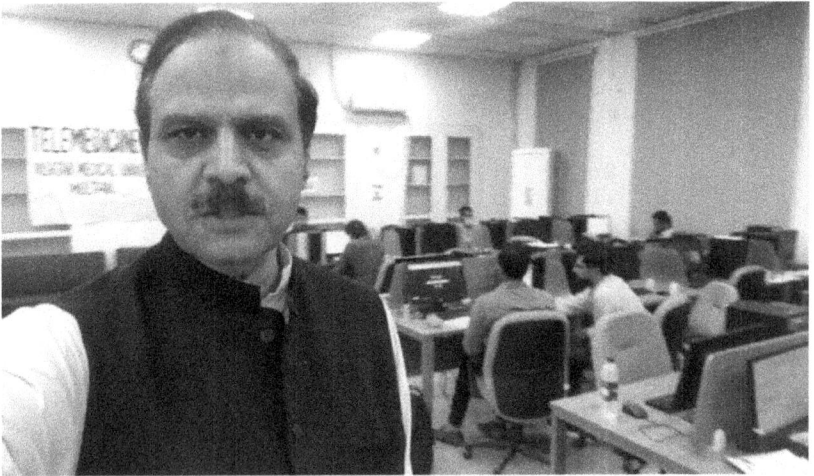

COVID-19 heroes remembered with "Wall of Heroes" in the Punjab Governor's House

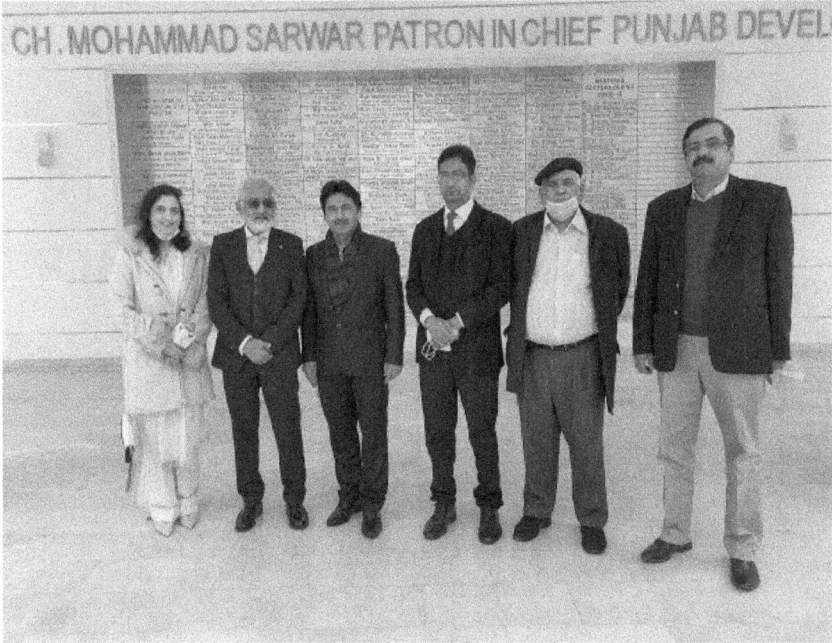

Punjab Governor Chaudhry Mohammad Sarwar paid tribute to the COVID-19 pandemic Heroes who lost their lives in the line of duty by laying the foundation of the "Wall of Heroes" in the Governor's House, Lahore. President, Dr Arif Alvi inaugurated the project and made special mention of the healthcare workers who lost their lives during the pandemic.

About the Authors

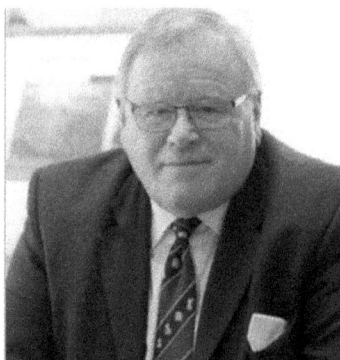

Prof (WILLIAM) ANGUS WALLACE
FRCS(Ed & Eng), FRCSEd(Orth), FFCI(UK), FFSEM(UK)

QUALIFICATIONS

MB ChB University of St Andrews (1972)

FRCS(Ed)   Royal College of Surgeons of Edinburgh (1977)

FRCSEd(Orth)   Royal College of Surgeons of Edinburgh (1985)

FRCS(Eng)   Royal College of Surgeons of England (1996)

Corresponding Fellow, American Shoulder & Elbow Surgeons (ASES - 1996)

Foundation Fellow of the Faculty of Sport and Exercise Medicine (FFSEM - 2006)

Foundation Fellow of the Faculty of Clinical Informatics UK (FFFCI UK – 2017)

Angus set up the Faculty of Health Informatics at the Royal College of Surgeons of Edinburgh in 2000 where he launched the first master's degree in health informatics, initially with the University of Bath and subsequently with the University of Edinburgh. During his five-year appointment as Dean of the Faculty of Health Informatics, he headed the team that developed the UK Surgical Electronic Logbook now used by all Trainee and Consultant surgeons in the UK to document their operations during training which has ensured good quality control of surgical training. He is passionate about delivering high volume, high-quality surgery through the NHS and has worked very hard in his own unit and, through his Regional Director work with RCS Eng, to make the NHS more efficient and productive.

In 2011, after 17 meetings at Nottingham University Hospitals and negotiations with the Orthopaedic Business Manager (Will Monaghan), the Corporate Operations Manager (John Peach), the Information Governance Manager (Rory King), and the PCT Service Change Group (Dr Hugh Porter) he set up his first NHS Telemedicine Clinic using the Cisco Webex platform in April 2011.

PRIZES, PRESTIGIOUS APPOINTMENTS & HONORARY AWARDS

- *Sir Walter Mercer Gold Medal (RCSEd) – Best Candidate in Orthopaedic Exam (1985)*
- *ABC Travelling Fellowship from the British Orthopaedic Association (1988)*
- *Honorary Fellowship British Orthopaedic Trainees Association (1990>)*
- *Honorary Membership Hellenic Ass of Orthopaedic Surgery & Traumatology (1995>)*
- *Weigelt-Wallace Award for exceptional medical care from the University of Texas (1995)*
- *Vice-President, Royal College of Surgeons of Edinburgh (1997-2000)*
- *Dean, Faculty of Health Informatics, Royal College of Surgeons of Edinburgh (2000-2005)*
- *Honorary Member of the British Indian Orthopaedic Society BIOS (2005>)*
- *Advisory Committee on Clinical Excellence Awards (ACCEA) Platinum Award (2005-15)*
- *Honorary Fellowship, Hong Kong College of Orthopaedic Surgeons (FHKCOS(Hon) 2011)*
- *Honorary Fellowship, Magyar Ortopéd Társaság, (FMOT(Hon) 2011)*
- *Sir Walter Mercer Gold Medal (RCS Ed) for the Walter Mercer Memorial Lecture (2015)*
- *The Codman Lecturer – the most prestigious Shoulder & Elbow Lecture presented at the 13th International Congress of Shoulder*

& Elbow Surgery, Korea (2016) Honorary Member, British Elbow & Shoulder Society (2016> one of 6 with only 3 still alive)

- *Honorary Fellowship, British Orthopaedic Association*
- *Honorary Fellowship, Faculty of Sport and Exercise Medicine (2017>)*
- *Foundation Fellow, Faculty of Clinical Informatics UK (2017)*
- *Pioneer Shoulder & Elbow Surgeon, Int Board of Shoulder & Elbow Surgery Award (2019)*

Dr SUHAIL CHUGHTAI FRCS

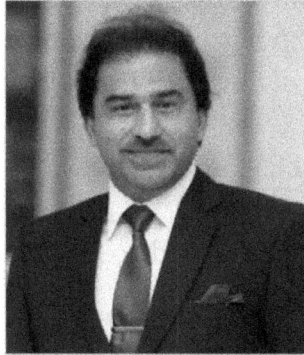

QUALIFICATIONS

MBBS	*Allama Iqbal Medical College, Lahore, Pakistan*
FRCS	*Fellowship in Surgery, Royal College of Physicians &*
	Surgeons, Glasgow, UK
MOUS	*Microsoft Certified Specialist (USA)*
FFLM	*Member, Faculty of Forensic and Legal Medicine, UK*
	eHealth Certification in e-Health - Sydney University, Australia

In progress - Masters in e-Health Management & Telemedicine - University of Rome, Italy

Dr Suhail Chughtai, is an orthopaedic surgeon with over 20 years of consultant level experience in the UK, Saudi Arabia and Pakistan. He felt there was a need for doctors to adapt to an increasingly technical, digitised world. This prompted him to study Computer Software and Hardware, receiving a Microsoft Specialist certification in 2001, and then going on to teach Medical IT across the globe. After taking a particular interest in Telemedicine as a vital bridge between the patient and the doctor, Dr Chughtai founded Medical City Online, a Telehealth Firm in the UK, which has designed over 20 International Telehealth and Medical IT projects. Part of this new approach views patients Telemedicine Software as "solutions", rather than just products, and the firm has been actively engaged in helping to lessen the impact of Covid-19 in Pakistan

PROFESSIONAL ROLES

- Orthopaedic Surgeon & Medico.legal Examiner, Harley Street, London, UK
- International Telehealth Expert, Telemedicine Software Designer/Instructor
- Lead Faculty of Health Informatics & Telehealth, Univ of Health Sciences, Pakistan

Chairman

- Medical City Online, London, UK (Telehealth Software and Consulting Firm)
- M L Professionals, London, UK (Business Medico-Legal Examination Firm)
- Pan Arab Telemedicine & Artificial Intelligence Conference 2019, UAE

Director Digital Health & Telemedicine for various organizations

- Association of Pakistani Physicians & Surgeons UK
- Adam Global Healthcare Division, UAE

AWARDS & RECOGNITION

Innovation in Telemedicine Software - By APPNA (USA)
Changing Lives of People by Telemedicine - By World Peace & Prosperity Foundation, UK

- Commonwealth Award for Innovative Software for Telemedicine and Online Education
- Ambassador: Patientory Association, Atlanta, USA (Healthcare Blockchain Firm)

Awards/Recognition for Setting up COVID-19 Pandemic Telemedicine Helpline

- Foreign Minister Honours, by Govt of Pakistan
- Governor Punjab Honours, Pakistan
- British Pakistani Foundation, UK
- Association of Pakistani Physician & Surgeons, UK
- University of Health Sciences, Pakistan
- Ravian's Society, GC University, Pakistan
- Allama Iqbal Medical College Alumni, UK

Chapter Authors

Prof Dr Javed Akram

Associate Prof Dr Somia Iqtadar

Captain(R) Muhammad Usman

Mr Jonathan M Fuchs

Dr Shehla Javed

Dr Rana Jawad Asghar

Mr Saflain Haider

Miss Jumel Grace Ola

*Career Profiles of the Chapter authors are shared
at the end of their contributed chapter.*

Acknowledgements

Several organisations have noted and acknowledged the effort by Medical City Online in conjunction with the relevant Pakistan Authorities such as teams from the University of Health Sciences, the Governor Punjab Team and the Citrus Telemedicine Team.

The list of organisations below duly recognised the value of work for Doctors 24/7 Online Telemedicine Helpline for COVID-19, either by referring to them on their websites or in different events or TV programs. We, the authors of the book, are thankful for their fervent support.

Faculty of Clinical Information, United Kingdom

Pakistan High Commission, United Kingdom

Foreign Office, Islamabad, Pakistan

Conversative Friends of Pakistan, United Kingdom

Primary and Secondary Health Department,

Punjab, Pakistan

Association of Pakistani Physicians & Surgeons,

UK – APPS UK

Akhuwat Foundation, Pakistan

British Pakistani Foundation, UK

Government College University Lahore, Pakistan

Association of Physicians of Pakistan Origin of North America – APPNA

Adam Global, Healthcare Division, UAE

World Congress of Overseas Pakistanis – WCOP – UK

Doctorscon – Premier Family Medical Organization in Pakistan

Alumni of Allama Iqbal Medical College, UK

World Union of Wound Healing Societies, UAE

Academy of Family Physicians of Pakistan

College of Family Medicine, Pakistan

International Inter-Professional Wound Care Group, UAE

Pakistan Society of Internal Medicine, Pakistan

Women Chamber of Commerce, Pakistan

Pakistan Poverty Alleviation Fund

Telemedicine Helpline, featured by major national TV channels

BBC England - Voice of America (Pak) - Geo TV Pak - Duniya TV Pak

Pointing your phone camera on the QR code will connect you to the video clip below, provided you do it through any QR reader app available free from the app store.

BBC World News reports Telemedicine Services in Pakistan setup by Dr Suhail Chughtai, arranging Virtual Teleward Rounds by UK Specialists through a special Telemedicine software to help patients in Corona ICU wards in Pakistani Hospitals.

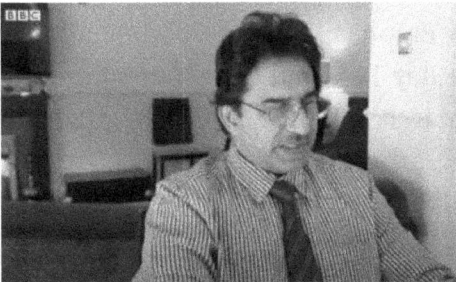

https://www.youtube.com/watch?v=9KP_yKR8VT0

Prof Angus Wallace at BBC East Midlands Channel gives a prelude on Telemedicine's role in fighting a Pandemic, exemplifying www.Doctors247.online as a model software for the purpose

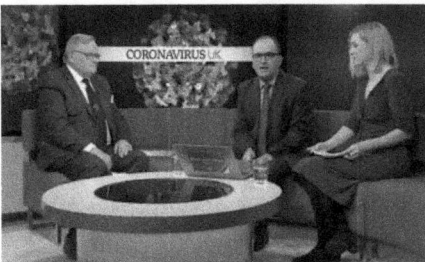

https://youtu.be/PbMGC1zGMh4

Dr Humayun Baig and Dr Farwah Rubab walk through the Telemedicine Helpline Hub setup at University of Health Sciences, Lahore in a short interview at TV Channel of Voice of America, Pakistan.

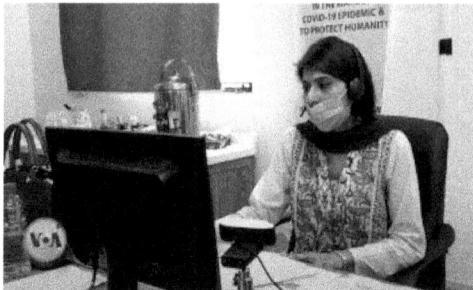

https://youtu.be/3VVhnWBlvIA

Dr Suhail Chughtai places emphasis on role of Telemedicine in fight against Covid, on the day Pakistan Government announced the Lockdown on 12th March 2020 at one of the largest TV networks of the country.

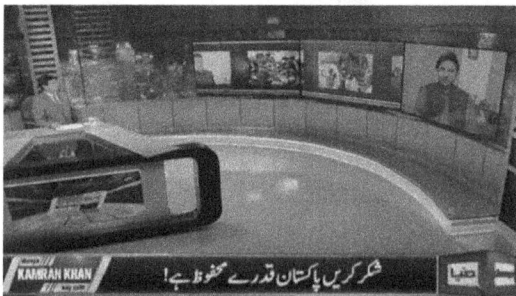

https://youtu.be/kynJj53qdrY?t=4140

Role of Telemedicine in the fight against Covid was emphasized on the day Pakistan Government announced the Lockdown on 25th March 2020 at one of the largest TV networks of the country.

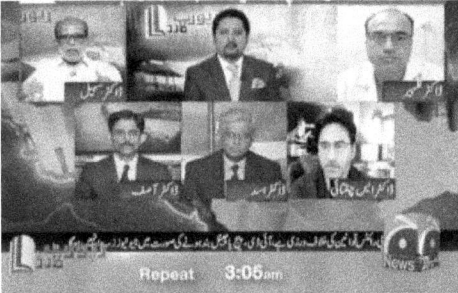

https://youtu.be/X17mFJTjTEc?t=543

You can view additional Press and Media reports about the Telemedicine Helpline setup on the website www.Doctors247.online

Chapter One

The Meeting of Two Minds

Authors: *Prof Angus Wallace & Dr Suhail Chughtai*

This book tells a unique story of two doctors who coincidentally happen to be Orthopaedic Surgeons, and had separately developed a passion for delivering care through Telemedicine technology. Suhail Chughtai developed an in-depth interest in technology while working as an Orthopaedic Surgeon in London. Angus Wallace set up an NHS Telemedicine service at Nottingham University Hospital in 2011 and became committed to delivering a Telemedicine service after that. Suhail and Angus have worked virtually, collaboratively, and symbiotically since late 2019 and have only had one face-to-face meeting in London, on 3rd March 2020.

We have summarised our professional careers in this chapter. Suhail Chughtai was a Pakistan born, but UK trained Orthopaedic Surgeon who developed higher skills in medical software designing and Angus Wallace was initially from Scotland but subsequently trained in England as an Orthopaedic Surgeon with an academic background but with a special interest in Medical Informatics for over 20 years.

Here, we share our individual paths of development before we came together through email communications in September 2019 and met in London on 3rd March 2020 to initiate a combined trek on the road of Telemedicine.

Suhail Chughtai's Journey
As an Orthopaedic Surgeon

Suhail, born in Pakistan, completed his medical graduation from Allama Iqbal Medical College, Lahore, Pakistan and completed his surgical fellowship from the Royal College of Physicians & Surgeons Glasgow, UK in 1993. He was an Orthopaedic Trainee in the UK from 1989 till 1995 which included his Higher Specialist Orthopaedic Training Rotational Program. He was appointed to a Locum Consultant Orthopaedic Surgeon's position in his early thirties in Scotland for a year before returning to Lahore, Pakistan in 1996.

Suhail continued his orthopaedic career in Pakistan for four years as a Consultant Orthopaedic Surgeon while he also served as an Assistant Professor in Orthopaedics (Hon) at Fatima Jinnah Medical College, Pakistan till 1999. He was later appointed in Saudi Arabia as a Consultant Orthopaedic Surgeon rotating between both the Ministry of Health and the Ministry of Defence for a further four years. In 2004, Suhail resumed his service with the NHS in the UK, taking up a Locum Consultant Orthopaedic Surgeon position.

Towards 2010, he additionally developed his Orthopaedic Injury Medico-legal Evaluation practice with around 20 medical examination venues across England, having a clinical base in Harley Street London, while being a member of the Faculty of Forensic & Legal Medicine UK.

As a Telehealth, Medical Technology Expert and Techpreneur

Suhail developed a deep and passionate interest in Medical IT during his early surgical career and effectively self-trained himself to be a Microsoft Certified Specialist since 2001. Subsequently, he acquired training and certification as a Microsoft Access Database Expert during his Orthopaedic practice in the UK. He has also recently completed his certification in e-Health Management from the University of Sydney. He is currently studying for his master's degree course in Telemedicine alongside his professional roles and responsibilities.

He was a regular Medical IT Instructor at Health Asia Conferences from 2001 onwards. He is the Founding Chairman of Medical City Online, a Telehealth Consulting and Software company based in the UK with connecting offices in several countries through the company's international Telehealth Business Associates.

Suhail is the lead Telehealth Software Architect for Medical City Online, supported by a large team of Web Developers working on his multiple Telehealth projects. He has designed over 20 Medical Software Projects, the majority being proprietary Medical City Online's Telehealth Projects that are currently deployed by private and government organisations in several countries.

He has instructed workshops, given lectures and been a keynote speaker at over 100 medical computing conferences since 2000 in the USA, UK, Germany, Pakistan, United Arab Emirates (UAE) and Saudi Arabia.

Suhail has regularly taught on various aspects of Telehealth subjects for over ten years with a range of topics covering both Clinical and Business sectors. Several of his courses and his training materials have been granted Continuous Medical Education accreditation, the most recent being at the University of Health Sciences, Lahore, Pakistan where he serves as Lead of the International Faculty for the master's degree course on Telehealth subjects.

His passion for sharing his skills and building the capacity of healthcare professionals has resulted in his regular invitations to large conferences like the Pan Arab Telemedicine Conference 2019 in UAE where he was appointed as the Conference Chairman at the two-day event with around 30 speakers from several countries.

Awards and Recognition in the field of Telehealth

Suhail received international recognition for his work on setting up the national Telemedicine Helpline in the fight against COVID-19 Pandemic in Pakistan not only by the Foreign Minister Honours Office and Governor Punjab Secretariate but also from the British Pakistani Foundation, UK, the Association of Pakistani Physician & Surgeons, UK, the University of Health Sciences, Pakistan, the Ravian's Society, the GC University, Pakistan and the Alumni Allama Iqbal Medical College, UK.

Various other awards include "Changing Lives of People through Telemedicine" presented by the World Peace & Prosperity Foundation, UK, "Innovative Software for Telemedicine and Online Education" by the Commonwealth Awards, "Innovation in Telemedicine Software" by APPNA (USA), and the "White Swan Award" for the creation of Digital TV (TVapex) for facilitating multi-cultural harmony in the UK.

Recent Contribution to the Telehealth related Literature

- ***Wallace WA, Chughtai S***: *Telemedicine, a Novel Way to Fight a Pandemic, Success Story from Pakistan. Book Author*
- ***Chughtai S:*** *Healthcare Services over Internet to revolutionize Pakistan Healthcare System. Pakistan Orthopaedic Association, volume 3, 2017*
- ***Chughtai S, Ellahham S:*** *Telemedicine to revolutionize outpatient-based healthcare. The Arab Hospital Magazine, January-February 2018, page 56*
- ***A.N Saigal, Chughtai S:*** *Telemedicine for Orthopaedic Consultations. The Musculoskeletal Journal of the Hospital for Special Surgery, New York*
- ***Chughtai S, Ellahham S:*** *Making Healthcare Facilities Available and Affordable using Telemedicine. The Arab Hospital Magazine, May-June 2018, page 18*
- ***Chughtai S:*** *Tele-Arthroscopic Surgical Supervision to enhance Patient Safety. Journal of Sports Medicine & Doping Studies, Nov 2018*
- ***Baloch S, Chughtai S, Ellahham S:*** *Telemedicine for Wound Care Management. The Arab Hospital Magazine, Jan-Feb 2019, page 90*

Angus Wallace's Journey as an Orthopaedic Surgeon

A ngus was raised in Dundee, Scotland. He carried out his Medical degree initially in St Andrews and completed it in Dundee, qualifying with MBChB in 1972. He moved to Nottingham in 1973 to teach Anatomy at Nottingham University before embarking on his surgical training first in Nottingham and Derby and subsequently in Newcastle-upon-Tyne from 1975 to 1977. After passing his Fellowship examinations at the Royal College of Surgeons of Edinburgh in 1977, he returned to Nottingham to carry out his Higher Orthopaedic Training from 1977 to 1984. He was appointed to his first Consultant appointment in Manchester in May 1985, an appointment both as an NHS Consultant and as a Senior Lecturer (similar to Assistant Professor) at the University of Manchester.

As a University Academic and subsequently as Professor of Orthopaedic & Accident Surgery in Nottingham

In 1978 Angus was awarded a 1-year Training Research Fellow Fellowship in Nottingham by the Medical Research Council in which he studied the movements of the shoulder and acromio-clavicular joint during everyday activities. Based on this background he was subsequently appointed to a Clinical Lecturer/Senior Registrar position at Nottingham University in 1981 with Professor William Waugh during which, in 1983, he was appointed to a nine-month Research Fellowship at Toronto Western Hospital with Dr Murray Wiley and returned to Nottingham in November 1983. His next academic post was as Senior Lecturer in Manchester in 1984 working with Professor Charles Galasko. In that post, he had three roles – an NHS Consultant Orthopaedic Surgeon plus his academic role with the University of Manchester, but he also held an appointment as the Medical Director for the North-Western Orthotic Unit, Salford and was also appointed as Medical Advisor to the Department of Orthopaedic Mechanics at the University of Salford. In 1985 Angus was appointed as Professor of Orthopaedic & Accident Surgery in Nottingham at the age of 36, the second youngest Professor of Orthopaedics in the UK at the time of his appointment. He held this post for 30 years and has published with his research teams over 300 research papers, 60 Chapters and Proceedings papers and 10 books.

As a Medical Information Technology (IT) Expert

Angus was elected to the Council of the Royal College of Surgeons of Edinburgh (RCSEd) in 1990, and he was elected a Vice-President of the RCSEd in 1997. In 1999 he had already developed a considerable interest in programming and Information Technology having self-trained as a Fortran IV and Basic programmer while carrying out his shoulder research. He was very conscious of the need for healthcare workers to become more computer literate and persuaded the RCSEd to establish the first Faculty of Health Informatics in the UK in 2000. He was appointed Dean of the new Faculty in 2000 and held that position for five years. He established the first master's degree in Health Informatics, initially in partnership with Bath University and later with Edinburgh University. He was also a member of the team (including Lester Sher, Mike Reed, Paul Calvert and Andrew Lamb) who designed and produced the eLogbook now used by all surgeons in training and all surgical trainers in the UK and Ireland.

Subsequently, Angus served on the England National Clinical Reference Panel (NCRP) as the Choose and Book Lead representing Orthopaedics (2006/7) and was Chair of the National Specialty Reference Group for Connecting for Health (2007-2009).

In February 2011, after very protracted negotiations with the Nottingham University NHS Trust, Angus set up his own Shoulder Telemedicine Clinic at Nottingham City Hospital and started carrying out consultations using the Cisco Webex Video platform.

In 2016/2017 Angus supported Dr John Williams when the Faculty of Clinical Informatics was being set up and became a Foundation Fellow in 2017. He was subsequently appointed as Chair of the Events Organising Committee of the Faculty of Clinical Informatics UK (2019-22).

Angus held the post of Regional Advisor for the Royal College of Surgeons of England (RCS Eng) from 2014 to 2019. Because he believed that Telemedicine Clinics would improve the efficiency of the delivery of health care he set up and ran a Symposium with the RCS Eng on "Running and Setting up Virtual Surgical Outpatients Clinics" in May 2019. This was very successful and stimulated the setting up of even more Telemedicine clinics in the UK.

The Meeting of Minds – How it happened

Angus had taken over the organisation of the Faculty of Clinical Informatics First Scientific Conference planned for May 2020. He wanted to arrange an Instructional Course on "How do Virtual Clinics Work?" and needed a prominent International Speaker to showcase his Instructional Course. In September 2019 he sent the following email to Suhail Chughtai, and the subsequent email trail is shown below:

From: Prof Angus Wallace
Sent: 24 September 2019 18:00
To: Dr Suhail Chughtai, Telehealth Expert
Dear Dr Suhail Chughtai,
I would like to invite you to contribute to our Faculty of Clinical Informatics Conference scheduled for Thursday 14th May 2020 in London.

You can see from the attached draft programme that we are running early morning Instructional Courses.
You have given a number of interesting lectures on Telemedicine in the past. I wonder if you would be interested in running an early morning Instructional Course at our Conference on "The Challenges of running a Telemedicine Clinic".. ....

I look forward to hearing from you.

Angus Wallace
Chair, Conference Planning Committee, Faculty of Clinical Informatics

From: Dr Suhail Chughtai
Sent: 18 October 2019 19:26
To: Prof Angus Wallace
Subject: Participating in FCI Annual Scientific Conference 2020

Dear Prof,
It was a pleasure connecting with you.
I would be happy to contribute to the FCI Conference 2020 under the following heading:
Instructional Course 8 – How do Virtual Clinics Work?
Ideally, a 20-30 min would be suitable for an instructional presentation (including a demo video) though it can be packed in 15 min if need be.
I have been instructing day-long courses and hands-on Workshops for several years in various countries and contributing to your good work, will be an honour for me.
Best regards,
Suhail

From: Dr Suhail Chughtai
Sent: 12 February 2020 02:10
To: Prof Angus Wallace
Subject: Re: FW: Faculty of Clinical Informatics - Annual Scientific Conference - 14th May 2020
Dear Prof Wallace,
Hope you are well.
Recently, I was involved in two large Telehealth Conferences in UAE, being an organiser of the Pan Arab Telemedicine Conference, thus was behind communication with you. Will catch up now and will message soon to schedule a time for our conversation.
Best regards,
Suhail

Then the Coronavirus pandemic broke & Angus wrote the email below to the BBC

1st March 2020

From: Prof Angus Wallace
Sent: 01 March 2020 11:10
To: Hugh Pym (BBC); Rob Sissons (BBC East Midlands Today)
Cc: CHUGHTAI Suhail
Subject: Using modern technology to manage COVID-19

Dear Hugh and Rob,
Our NHS leaders are developing plans for dealing with COVID-19. Some of these are unrealistic and impractical.
I would like to offer some solutions using modern technology.
I set up a UK Shoulder Telemedicine Clinic in Nottingham in 2011 using Webex. My colleague Suhail Chughtai, based in London, runs his Telemedicine clinics internationally.
This is definitely the technology we should be using with this COVID-19 epidemic.

How would this help with the current epidemic?
1. Why are we moving all patients who test positive for COVID-19 into a hospital when over 80% do not have a serious illness?

Would we not be better to self-isolate in our own homes with monitoring being carried out centrally? This could be done by using your mobile phone for Telemedicine consultations and, centrally we could set up a COVID-19 monitoring centre with a twice a day Telemedicine consultation carried out by a nurse, doctor or healthcare support worker.

2. If the patient's condition deteriorates then they should be transferred to a hospital for intensive treatment, but this would reduce transfer to hospitals by 80%

3. Once the condition has resolved, we could arrange a deep clean of the patient's home.

4. The location of the self-isolating patient could be monitored using the "Find my friends" or similar Apps to ensure that the patient remains in their own home.

The option of self-isolation is likely to be very attractive to most patients.

My colleague Suhail Chughtai has the technology to monitor the patient's temperature remotely, and we have developed methods for examining patients remotely. Please pass on this suggestion if you feel it is worthwhile and might be considered by those developing plans at present.
Angus

From: Prof Angus Wallace Sent: 01 March 2020 07:39
To: CHUGHTAI Suhail
Subject: Coronavirus - An Opportunity for Telemedicine

Suhail, The Coronavirus Epidemic is a golden opportunity to highlight how valuable Telemedicine Clinics could be for the NHS. Could we work together to support the NHS at this crucial time?
Angus

2nd March 2020

From: Dr Suhail Chughtai <director@medicalcity.online>
Sent: 02 March 2020 10:27
To: Prof Angus Wallace
Subject: Re: Coronavirus - An Opportunity for Telemedicine

Dear Prof,
You are spot-on, e.g., I got a few calls from conferences happening in UAE where they are now going to use my e-Classroom for connecting with Speakers. Also, for Teleconsultations, last Friday, I created two Online Medical Boards for some VIP patients in Pakistan and India, who now are reluctant to travel and prefer to rely on Telemedicine.

Let's connect and discuss. I am in London at St. Mary's College where a similar project is being discussed as the Vice-Chancellor of Univ of Health Sciences in Pakistan is visiting.
If you are in London tomorrow (3rd March around 12 midday in Central London, I can mediate a meeting between you and the VC). I am helping to provide Teleconsult Tech and Online Classroom for this rather large project. If you are free today, please message via text and I shall respond to share more.
Regards,
Suhail

4th March 2020

From: Dr Suhail Chughtai
Sent: 04 March 2020 08:54 To: Prof Angus Wallace
Cc: Hugh.Pym; SISSONS Rob(BBC_EastMidlands);
MONAGHAN Will(NHSX)

Subject: Re: Using modern technology to manage COVID-19

Dear Prof Wallace,
Telemedicine is shifting the paradigm of healthcare by adding a strong element of remote care.
My work over the last decade being a medical professional and software technologist is focussed on developing a Clinic-like Interface for Telemedicine. I believe that Video Conferencing is only part of Telemedicine and to give a patient near-real feel of an in-person Teleconsult, the design and interface of Telemedicine matters.

I would be able to elaborate more soon on a demo.
Regards, Suhail

BBC UK highlights the usefulness of Telemedicine in remote care during COVID pandemic

Rob Sissons at BBC East Midlands Today responded to my email of 1st March, and we arranged some BBC filming of a Telemedicine Consultation carried out at my home just outside Nottingham at lunchtime on Wednesday 4th March. I subsequently carried out a BBC interview with Dominic Heale in the Nottingham BBC Studio at 18.30 on 4th March that is now available via this link.

Just before the BBC interview, Angus visited London on 3rd March 2020 and met up with Professor Javed Akram as detailed in Chapter 2.

Angus's plan to help the NHS in the UK as depicted in his email to Hugh Pym and Rob Sissons on 1st March became re-directed to Pakistan by Suhail Chughtai and formed the basis of the achievements listed later in this book.

How the Coronavirus Pandemic unfolded – Angus Wallace's personal experience.

On 27th February the UK Government had announced that a "New surveillance system for early detection of COVID-19" had been launched. On 2nd March the BBC reported "Corona virus: Widespread transmission in UK 'highly likely'"

Following his BBC East Midlands Interview on 4th March Angus tried to communicate with NHS leaders in the UK to encourage the use of Telemedicine consultations to triage patients to no avail. Both his wife Jackie and Angus became increasingly concerned about the pandemic.

On 11th March, NHS England announced that testing in NHS laboratories would increase from testing 1,500 to 10,000 per day [3], the same day that the Liverpool v Atletico Madrid soccer match took place in Liverpool. This was particularly worrying because the Corona virus pandemic was overwhelming medical services in Northern Italy at that time, and it had become clear that the Corona virus disease was very infectious. At the same time, the first major horse racing event of the year – the Cheltenham Festival in Cheltenham, Gloucestershire took place from 10th-13th March 2020. It was surprising that this went ahead when NHS England had already decided to increase Coronavirus testing.

Jackie and Angus's daughter Suzanne (a Consultant Obstetrician) and her husband Daren Forward (a Consultant Trauma Surgeon) both worked at Nottingham University Hospitals, and both were watching the pandemic unfolding in their hospitals. Jackie and Angus were instructed by them to self-isolate from 13th March 2020 which they did religiously until 12th July when their first venture from their home was when they joined friends who were celebrating their 50th wedding anniversary with drinks in their garden – a celebration carried out with six people all together but with appropriate social-distancing.

The official England national lock-down was declared on 23rd March 2020, 10 days after Jackie and Angus had started their personal lockdown period.

From 13th March Jackie and Angus remained isolated, but Angus continued to work remotely, with some of his work devoted to the activities highlighted in the subsequent chapters in this book.

The Faculty of Clinical Informatics decided to commence a webinar programme in late March 2020 and Angus offered to run the first webinar on "The Potential Role of Virtual Clinics during the COVID-19 Pandemic" on 3rd April 2020 using MS Teams. This one-hour webinar included 10-minute presentations from Angus on "Experience with a Shoulder Telemedicine Clinic in Nottingham" and from Suhail on "Setting up a Telemedicine Platform in Pakistan". This webinar is available via the QR code.

Although this webinar was well-received, Angus was unable to progress his guidance through the various NHS channels that were available to him.

Chapter Two

The University of Health Sciences, Lahore connection

Authors: Prof W Angus Wallace & Dr Suhail Chughtai

3rd March 2020

On Tuesday 3rd March 2020, Professor Javed Akram, Vice-Chancellor (VC) of the University of Health Sciences (UHS), Lahore, with his wife, Dr Shehla Javed (Chief Executive of Don Valley Pharmaceuticals, Founder President of the Women Chamber of Commerce and CEO of Akram Medical Complex, Lahore) were visiting London to discuss with the Academic Council of the "Queen Mary's Medical & Dental College, London" future academic collaboration with the UHS. A meeting with Prof Angus Wallace in the cafeteria of the Royal College of Physicians, next to Regent's Park, London was set up by Suhail Chughtai who had known Prof Akram and his wife Dr Shehla Javed for several years. The aim of the meeting was to explore a collaboration between UHS, Suhail Chughtai, and Angus Wallace in relation to developing a master's degree in Telemedicine at UHS in Lahore.

Professor Akram being a very forward-looking VC realised that, with increasing uptake of Telemedicine practice in Pakistan, there would be a need for an increasingly sophisticated training programme for both those running the Telemedicine platforms and those delivering a Telemedicine service.

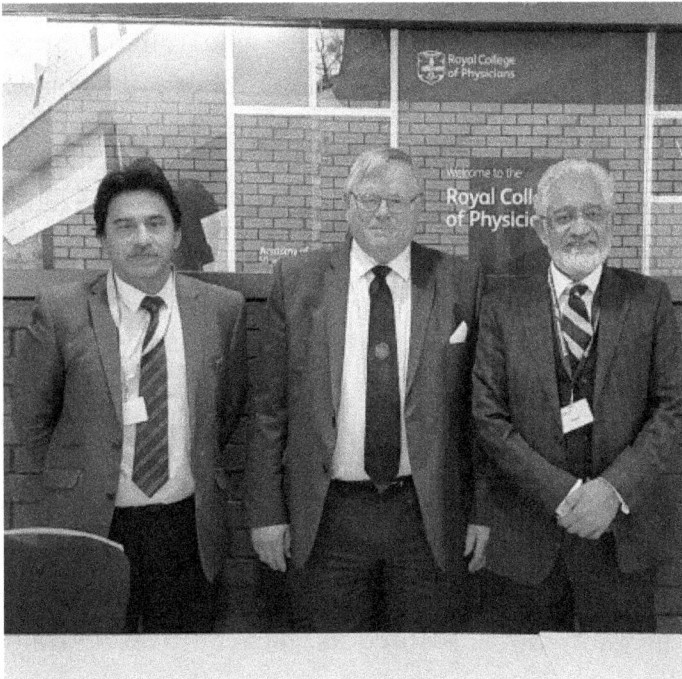

Suhail had developed his own Telehealth Software and Consulting Company (Medical City Online) in London and had been delivering Telemedicine Consultations for a number of years. Angus had set up an approved NHS Telemedicine Clinic at the Nottingham University Hospitals using the Cisco Webex platform in 2011. Together Suhail and Angus had the knowledge and skills to help UHS while Prof Akram was eager to benefit from the combined expertise of both experts. He agreed at our meeting to fast track the appointment of both Suhail Chughtai as an Adjuvant Professor at the UHS, working predominantly virtually from London and Angus Wallace, working virtually from Nottingham as Head of Health Informatics, in a newly created Department of Health Informatics, Telehealth and Artificial Intelligence at the UHS. These appointments were subsequently made in May 2020 after the approval of the department came through in the UHS Board of Governor's Meeting in early April 2020.

Over the following week, Angus Wallace was able to contact the Course Administrator who ran his previous master's degree course at the Royal College of Surgeons of Edinburgh (RCSEd), Alice Breton. Alice actually lives in New Zealand and had coordinated the master's degree course in Health Informatics in Edinburgh (RCSEd) Scotland virtually from her home in New Zealand. Fortuitously the RCSEd Health Informatics course had been closed down in 2015 because it was not considered mainstream surgical training. Alice Breton was then appointed Education Lead for the RCSEd, responsible for two postgraduate diplomas at RCSEd one on "Remote and Offshore Medicine (online)" and one on "Mountain Medicine (online and in the field)" before being offered redundancy in September 2019. The opportunity for her to reactivate her duties in Pakistan was appealing, and she was duly appointed as master's degree Graduate Coordinator.

Alice started her work for UHS in May 2020, and the different modules of the master's degree Course were decided in June and July 2020. Over the same period, Angus attempted to encourage collaborative parallel courses in the UK. Because of the Coronavirus pandemic, the UK was effectively shut-down, and no progress could be made despite contacts being attempted with Liverpool University, Bradford University, Newcastle-upon-Tyne University and Cambridge University.

One of the urgent requirements of the UHS was to set up a Certificate level course to facilitate the training of the volunteers who were offering to help with the Corona Telemedicine service for the COVID-19 crisis. Suhail worked night and day to create an eight-lecture programme for the Certificate course delivered online between 9th May and 7th June.

Most of the teaching was carried out virtually from the UK, but some local lecturers from Pakistan were also included.

Relevant email trail below from 1st March 2020

From: Prof Angus Wallace   Sent: 01 March 2020 07:39
To: CHUGHTAI Suhail (MedicalCity); MONAGHAN Will (NHSX)
Subject: Coronavirus - An Opportunity for Telemedicine

Suhail, The Coronavirus Epidemic is a golden opportunity to highlight how valuable Telemedicine Clinics could be for the NHS. Could we work together to support the NHS at this crucial time? I set up my first Telemedicine Clinic with Will Monaghan, who is now working for NHSX. Will, I know that Suhail and I understand the technology and can make it work. Can we do anything to help?
Angus

From: Dr Suhail Chughtai   Sent: 03 March 2020 08:10
To: Prof Angus Wallace; Prof Javed Akram
Subject: Re: Coronavirus - An Opportunity for Telemedicine

Dear Professor Angus Wallace,
Thank you for the information.
We can be at the Royal College of Physicians (Regent's Park) and wait for you at 1:30 pm. Our commitment at St. Mary's Hospital will be over by 1:00 pm, and we shall move to RCP.
The Cafeteria of RCP may be a place to meet and have tea together with the Vice-Chancellor of the University of Health Sciences, Pakistan. This university has academic jurisdiction over 56 Medical Colleges of Pakistan and Prof Javed Akram, being its VC is keen to develop external Medical IT links.
Please confirm if you are able to join us at RCP at 1:30 pm today for tea and a 30-45 min chat.
Thank you   Suhail Chughtai

Meeting with Prof Javed Akram (Vice-Chancellor, University of Health Sciences (UHS), Pakistan), 3rd March 2020, Royal College of Physicians, Regents Park, London NW1 4LE

Angus met Prof Javed Akram (VC UHS), Dr Shehla Javed (Chief Executive of Don Valley Pharmaceuticals, Founder President of the Women Chamber of Commerce, Past High Commissioner for Pakistan) who were invited by Dr Suhail Chughtai (Founder & Project Director of Medical City Online) to discuss 2-year MSc Programme for UHS (1-hour meeting).

From: Prof Angus Wallace
Sent: 05 March 2020 10:55
To: Prof Javed Akram; Shehla Akram
Cc: CHUGHTAI Suhail; BRETON Alice (Home)
Subject: Progressing a 2-year MSc in Biomedical Informatics in Pakistan

Dear Professor Akram,
It was good to meet you on Tuesday. As requested, I am attaching my CVs. One covers the period up to 2015 when I officially retired, and one covers 2015-2020 and highlights my activities since retirement.
I have also included the Health Education England Topol review that is directly relevant to our discussions and describes the recommended way forward that is now taking place in England.
When I set up the MSc in Health Informatics at the Royal College of Surgeons of Edinburgh (RCSEd) in 2000 (I was Dean of Health Informatics for five years), I appointed Alice Breton as our Course Coordinator.

Alice lives in New Zealand and ran the course from her home but with regular trips to Edinburgh for one week MSc on-site courses. In September 2019 the Royal College of Surgeons of Edinburgh decided that they no longer wished to run Health Informatics and Alice was

made redundant. I have spoken to her on Skype today, and she would
be very interested in helping you with your new master's degree Course
on a part-time basis similar to how she worked with the RCSEd. If you
felt this was something you wished to do, I would be able to give her
an outstanding reference for the work she has done in the past 15
years with the RCSEd. Alice has told me she may be able to provide a
Curriculum template for us to work on, and I have also asked if she would
provide you with her CV for you to consider.

I look forward to our further discussions.
Angus

The First Telemedicine Course run at UHS on MS Teams

Prof Angus Wallace – UK   *09 May 9:30 pm, Saturday*
Dr Suhail Chughtai – UK

Introduction & History of Telemedicine - Types of Telemedicine – Setting up a Telemedicine practice? Software & Hardware requirements

Dr Suhail Chughtai – UK   *10 May 9:30 pm, Sunday*
Dr Sohaib Javed – Pak (Co-instructor)

**Anatomy of a Telemedicine Software - Basic Elements of a Telemedicine Software
Advanced Elements of a Telemedicine Software**

Dr Suhail Chughtai - UK   *16 May 9:30 pm, Saturday*

Applications of Telemedicine in day-to-day medical practice - Impact of Telemedicine on Healthcare Economy - Entrepreneurship in Telemedicine practice

Dr Suhail Chughtai – UK   *17 May 9:30 pm, Sunday*
Dr Ali Syed – Pak (Co-instructor)

Live Medical Tele-consultations: Benefits & Limits - Techniques of engaging a patient over Virtual Consultation - Physical Consultation vs Virtual Consultation

Prof Angus Wallace – UK   *30 May 9:30 pm, Saturday*

Telemedicine based Employee Healthcare - Telemedicine for Medical Research Medical Board Formation via Telemedicine Software

Dr Suhail Chughtai – UK   31 May 9:30 pm, Sunday
Dr Ahmed Ejaz – Pak (Co-instructor)

How to build patient's Electronic Medical Record - Using Telemedicine Software as a Practice Management Software - Medico-legal coverage for the doctors

 Dr Junaid Hassan (UK)   06 June 9:30 pm, Saturday
Dr Humayun Baig (Pak)

Setting up Specialist Telemedicine Clinics – Tele-physiotherapy & Tele-dentistry, Also, Tele-cardiology – Tele-dermatology – Tele-psychiatry and more

Dr Suhail Chughtai – UK   07 June 9:30 pm, Sunday
Dr Ahmed Ejaz – Pak (Co-instructor)

References

1.   *UK_Government, New surveillance system for early detection of COVID-19. 2020.*
        https://www.gov.uk/government/news/new-surveillance-system-for-early-detection-of-COVID-19

2.   *BBC_News, Coronavirus: Widespread transmission in UK 'highly likely'. 2020.*
        https://www.bbc.co.uk/news/uk-51700604

3.   *Health_Services_Journal (HSJ), Daily Insight: Budget day maths. 2020.*
        https://www.hsj.co.uk/daily-insight/daily-insight-budget-day-maths/7027096.article

Chapter Three

From Ground Zero to Doctors 24/7 Telemedicine Helpline

The Journey Summarised

Author: *Dr Suhail Chughtai*

The sequence of events
The challenges faced
The launch of the Telemedicine helpline on 18th March 2020
Expansion of the Telemedicine project to a national level
Raising public awareness about the service
Emerging stories out of the Telemedicine helpline

THE SEQUENCE OF EVENTS

12th March 2020, the idea shared

I was visiting Lahore, Pakistan to attend the annual conference of the Pakistan Society of Internal Medicine as a keynote speaker on the Telemedicine topic, "Revolutionizing Pak Healthcare through Telemedicine". The host organization's Secretary-General, Dr Somia Iqtadar, had invited me to join in at the opening day of the conference as one of the panel members to address the media at the press conference launch.

Upon arriving at the Lahore airport, on the night before the conference, I kept hearing people talk about the Corona epidemic with a sense of uncertainty and with speculation that the Corona epidemic situation in Pakistan might become similar to China and Iran which, being neighbouring countries, had significant people travelling into and out of both countries from Pakistan.

Those who knew me asked what will happen if the Corona epidemic goes out of control in Pakistan, how will we manage it considering the large population size and the poor availability of Intensive Care Beds and similar questions with a degree of fear of the unknown in their voice. The Medics appeared to be deeply concerned about the number of ventilators being insufficient to manage the chest and breathing-related advanced stage of the infection. People talked about China's strategy of winning the battle by using a strict lockdown, and they appeared concerned about how to reach a doctor during a lock-down which was then being considered by the Government.

I had an uneasy and short sleep that night as I kept thinking about people's questions and their sense of looming uncertainty. I woke up early in the morning to write down points of the plan that I had conceived through the night; "fighting COVID-19 epidemic with the help of a Telemedicine Helpline". I thought it would minimize the number of people visiting hospitals and clinics with non-urgent medical conditions, including mild to moderate symptoms of suspected Corona infection. To me, it seemed an effective means to limit people movement, yet making medical care available to them. The plan would suit the restrictions placed in case the Pakistan Government were to impose a lockdown, which was expected at any time.

While being driven to the Pearl Continental Hotel Lahore, the venue of the Press Conference launch, I was able to draft my thoughts about a project outline. I had a few minutes chat with Prof Dr Javed Akram and Prof Dr Aftab Mohsin who endorsed the concept and encouraged me to bring the idea out into the open at the Press Conference due to take place a few minutes later.

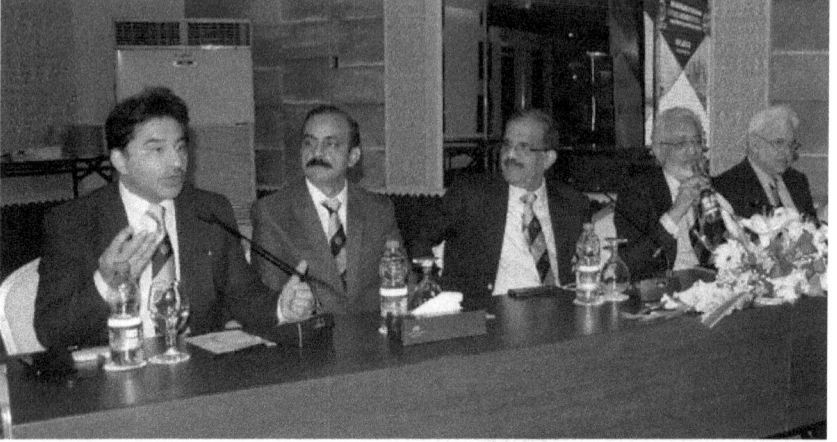

12th March 2020, Pak Society of Internal Medicine Launch Press Conference where Dr Suhail Chughtai introduced the idea of Telemedicine as a tool to assist fight Corona Pandemic.

As I presented the idea at the Press Conference, questions were raised, which reflected a lack of trust in Telemedicine for such a purpose; however, to some, it made sense. Looking back, I am glad that Prof Dr Javed Akram, Vice-Chancellor University of Health Sciences (UHS), exhibited true leadership qualities and without wasting any time, took further steps.

Prof Akram formed a team to help me set up a control and command centre for the Telemedicine Helpline at the University of Health Sciences premises.

Harnessing support from the Administrative and Political Machinery

13th March 2020

The very next day, the Pakistan Government announced an immediate lockdown, which resulted in a premature end of the PSIM Annual Medical Conference that I was attending. At this stage, Prof Dr Javed Akram thought it was the right moment to involve the relevant Punjab Government Authorities for a more comprehensive implementation of the Telemedicine Helpline to provide free medical advice to the public during the impending lock-down. The Governor of Punjab, Chaudhary Mohammad Sarwar was invited to become involved. He not only believed in the strength of the idea but also went a step further and provided political leadership, taking ownership of the responsibility for the necessary planning that was required and he responded fervently and aptly by calling an urgent meeting of the Vice-Chancellors of all the Medical Universities of Punjab to discuss an implementation plan for setting up a chain of Telemedicine Hubs all over the province which, with a population of 110 million, needed a massive infrastructure of medical professionals engaged for the purpose.

Setting arrangements in motion while working remotely from the UK

I was scheduled to fly back to the United Kingdom on 15th March, but as there was an impending lockdown taking place in the UK as well, I feared that I might not be able to fly and reach home if I delayed further.

14th March 2020

The night before leaving for the UK, I met the recently formed team members at the University Health Sciences, which included Dr Khurram Shahzad and Dr Humayun Taimoor, Mohammad Farhan, Asif Mehmood and others. We discussed the structure of the project for a quick implementation as the number of Corona positive cases were rising at a very fast pace in Pakistan.

15th March 2020

While I was waiting at the airport lounge to board the flight, I called an urgent telephone meeting with my relevant web developers to give them preliminary instructions to begin re-designing work on my existing Telemedicine software and wait for detailed instructions a few hours later.

16th March 2020

Upon landing at London Heathrow on the morning of 16th March, my team who had worked through the night gave me a demo of the draft design on my mobile phone, while I was in a taxi being driven home.

As I reached home, I resumed working with my Web Team who stayed up for 48 hours with few breaks. Everyone involved, including our Web and Mobile apps developers, Graphic Designers, Quality Analysts and Software Testers understood the importance of the time constrains and acted responsibly while working tirelessly on this fast tracked Telemedicine project.

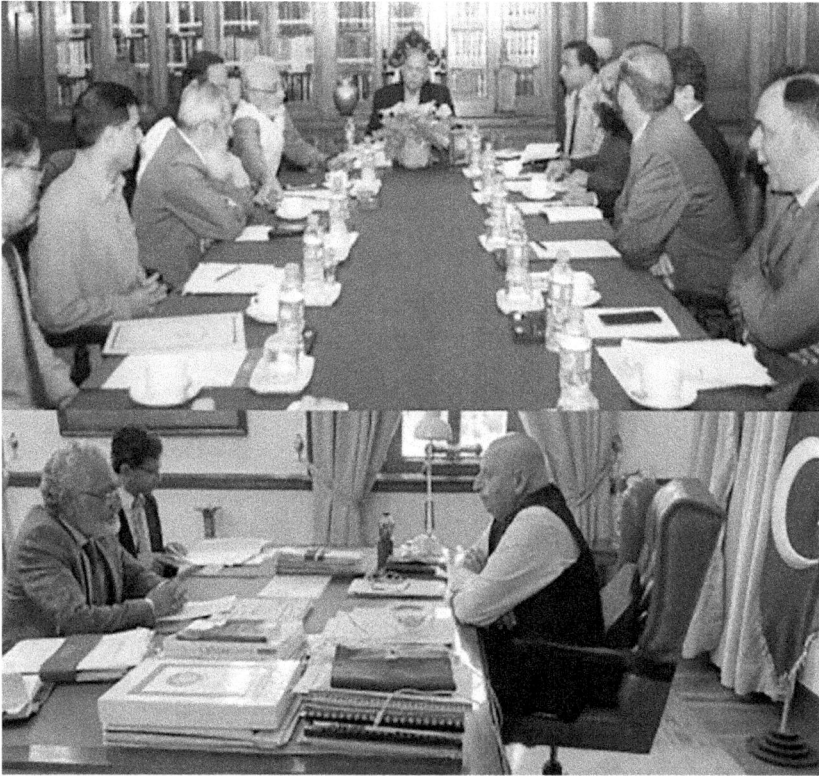

Chaudhary Muhammad Sarwar called for a grand meeting with Vice Chancellors of major Medical Universities in Punjab and then had one-on-one meeting with Prof Dr Javed Akram to initiate the formation of Central Telemedicine Hub at University of Health Sciences, to which other peripheral hubs would be linked via www.Doctors247.online.

THE CHALLENGES FACED

Given the time constraint and the nature of the project, we faced several challenges that threatened a timely deployment of the proposed Telemedicine Helpline.

A suitable Telemedicine Software for 24/7 Medical Teleconsultation Service

This was the major issue as there was no time for experimentation of technology. We needed a perfect Telemedicine solution to work right away with no technical hiccups with all the "ifs and buts" ironed out previously.

To keep Telemedicine safe and straightforward for both patients and doctors, I decided to modify one of my full featured Telemedicine Software by re-designing it to work like a Telemedicine Helpline. It was important to keep a bare-minimum Telemedicine service, yet suitable enough for healthcare delivery. Some features needed for a detailed Outpatient Consultation were removed to keep the Telemedicine Helpline function without the need to take an appointment. To make doctors readily connectible to the members of the public visiting the website on desktop, laptop computers or hand-held devices, the platform needed to be made flawless. I was of the view that a video consultation alone would not make it a totally effective virtual medical Teleconsultation. I thus incorporated a Corona-Scoring system, a simplified electronic medical record interface, clinical investigations and prescription writing module and also a patient education via images portal.

I worked on simplifying the existing electronic medical record system so that it would take photos of the available medical investigations such as ECG, X-rays etc., and it would upload the images via the device being used for the Teleconsultation. A follow-up module was also incorporated to ensure providing continuing medical care was as complete as possible through the online service.

One challenge was to keep it simple for the patients as, in Pakistan, online consultations were a relatively new concept, and there was a need to gain the public's trust. I attempted to create a quick and direct connecting interface between an online doctor and a patient using up to three screens at the doctor's end. The patient's record would be saved under the mobile phone number record; hence the same mobile phone holder could revisit for a follow-up Teleconsultation if needed.

The website was made mobile responsive thus the website, *www.Doctors247.online* was friendly towards handheld devices. Mobile Apps were also re-designed within 3-4 days to enhance the user's experience. All this meant engaging a team of 6-7 web and mobile Apps developers who worked almost 18 hours a day over two days to re-design the software and mobile apps, getting the Telemedicine Website, *www.Doctors247.online* and its relevant mobile Apps ready in just over two days.

The Deployment of a large number of doctors without salary

Getting a large number of doctors to take calls from all over the country meant having a large number of doctors available for consultations. There were no funds available, and it seemed a show-stopper but at this critical point, the Vice-Chancellor of the University of Health Sciences, Prof Dr Javed Akram came to the rescue by inviting young doctors to join the Telemedicine Helpline project in exchange for academic support to the volunteers. The call-out for volunteers attracted over 500 doctors contacting the University of Health Sciences office within two days making our job of creating a round-the-clock roster for doctors possible.

Training a large number of Doctors in a short span of time

I became involved in the Online Software Training remotely from the UK while the first set of doctors were trained face to face through small group meetings facilitated by Prof Nasir Shah, Head of Department of Family Medicine. Online sessions were arranged with the help of local facilitators, and I took the volunteering doctors through the steps of the process of a Teleconsultation again remotely.

Subsequently, I managed to train two master Trainers, Dr Sohaib Imtiaz and Mr Asif Mehmood who could take turns to continue transferring knowledge ending up training over 300 doctors in one week from the point the software was ready.

Hardware Logistics of setting up a Telemedicine Hub

The computer labs used for the Telemedicine Hubs were provided by the University of Health Sciences Lahore, Punjab which resolved a major issue of buying new equipment. The internet services, electricity, space, furniture, and security for the place was all managed by the University staff. At the same time, the arrangements for pick-and drop-off for female doctors along with the provision of food was taken care of by the University office under the direct instructions of the Vice-Chancellor, Prof Dr Javed Akram.

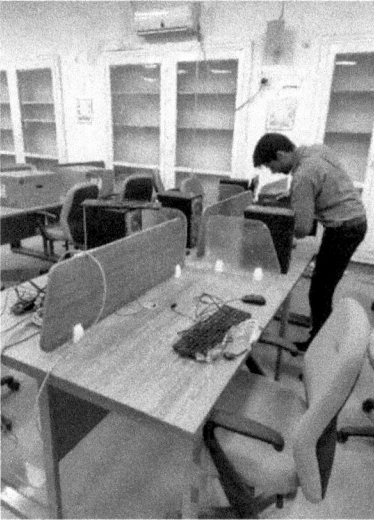

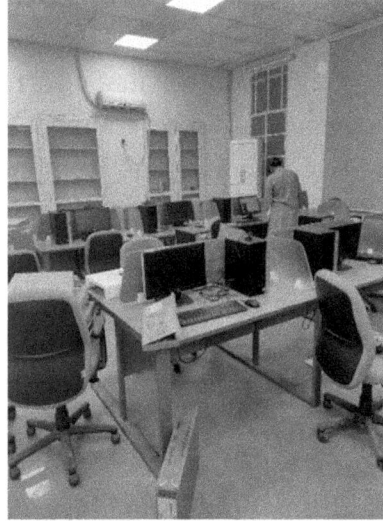

Central Telemedicine Hub at University of Health Sciences Lahore being setup overnight.

The Management Team for the Telemedicine Service 24/7

Dr Khurram Shahzad and Dr Humayun Taimoor took charge of the Administration and Operations putting their years of experience of project management into action, which helped not only put pieces of the puzzle together but articulated them into a flowing mechanism with ease and consistency.

The Launch of the Telemedicine Helpline
on 18th March 2020

The coordinated effort and passionate work by a quickly formed team spanning over two days finally took the shape of a Telemedicine Helpline project with www.Doctors247. online as the portal for Teleconsultations, supported by telephone lines as well for the backup. The website and the project were launched by the Governor of Punjab, Chaudhary Muhammad Sarwar at the University of Health Sciences, the location of the Command and Control Centre of the Telemedicine Helpline Service.

Dr Suhail Chughtai gave a briefing over a video link from England explaining the objectives to be achieved through the service. The inauguration was hosted by Prof Dr Javed Akram, the VC of Univ of Health Sciences while notable guests included Justice Tassadaq Jeelani (the Chair of Board of Governors of Univ of Health Sciences and former Chief Justice of Pakistan), Dr Rizwan Naseer (Director General of National Rescue Services 1122), Dr Amjad Saqib (Founder Director of Akhuwat, the largest Microfinance National Service) and several others from Lahore.

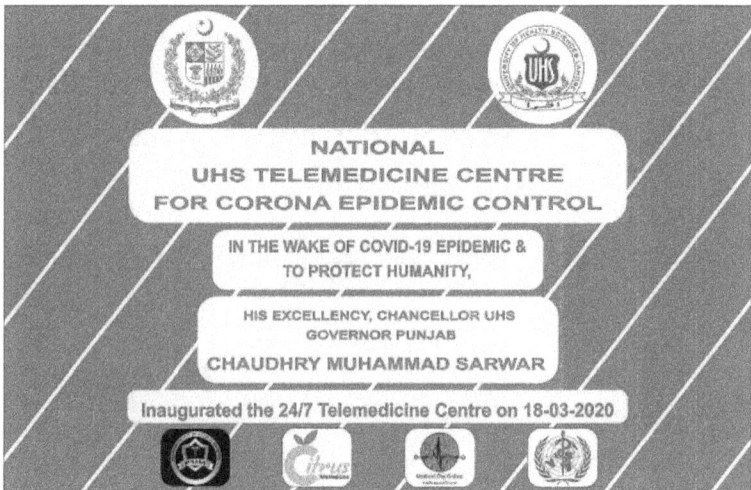

NATIONAL
UHS TELEMEDICINE CENTRE
FOR CORONA EPIDEMIC CONTROL

IN THE WAKE OF COVID-19 EPIDEMIC &
TO PROTECT HUMANITY,

HIS EXCELLENCY, CHANCELLOR UHS
GOVERNOR PUNJAB
CHAUDHRY MUHAMMAD SARWAR

Inaugurated the 24/7 Telemedicine Centre on 18-03-2020

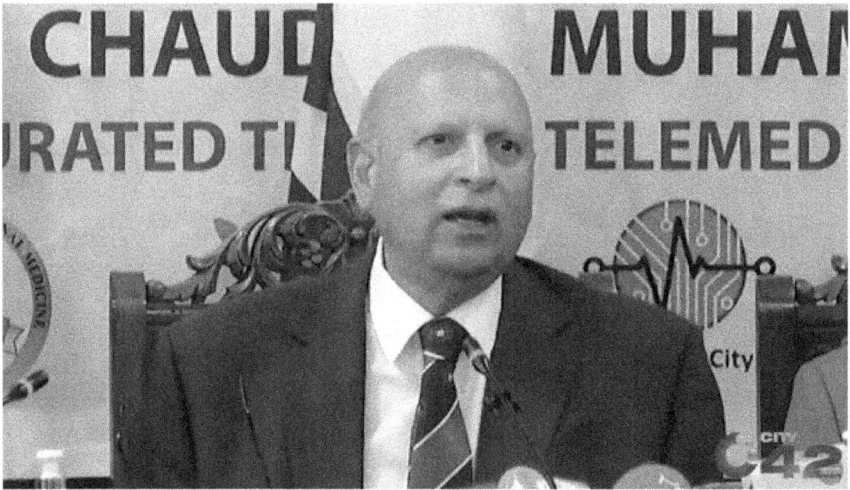

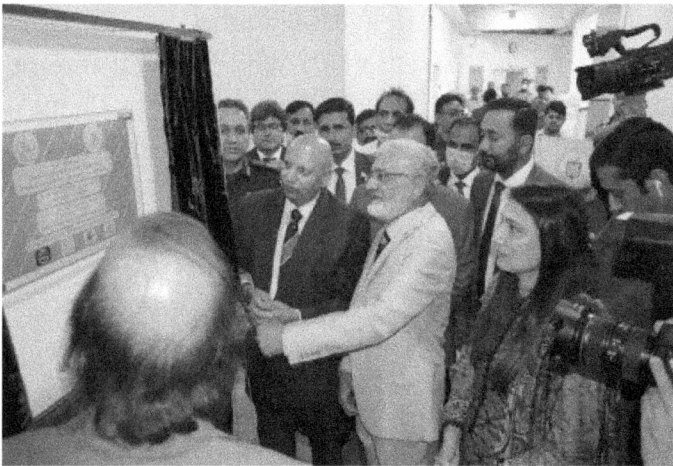

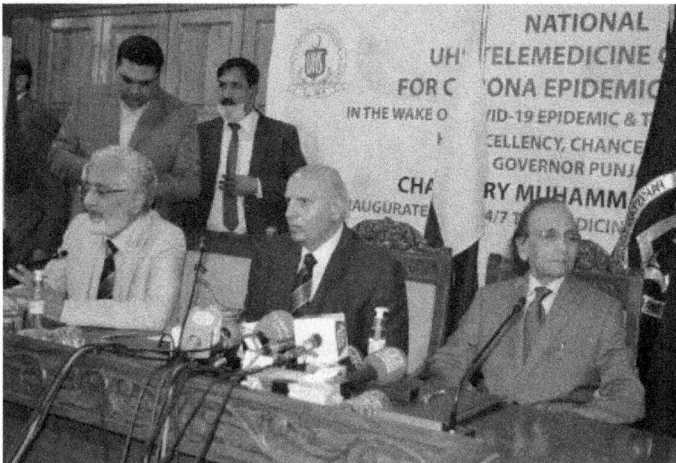

Expansion of the Telemedicine project to a National Level

Considering the impact of the Telemedicine helpline project, a chain of Telemedicine hubs was created at several medical universities and institutions in the province of Punjab. The Governor of Punjab offered fervent support and logistic assistance which was a great help since the team, led by Dr Shahzad and Dr Humayun, required this support while the lockdown restrictions were being imposed and they needed to reach other cities for setting up their Telemedicine hubs.

I was involved in delivering online training sessions at each of the hubs (remotely) while special interest was taken by the Governor of Punjab and the Vice-Chancellor of the University of Health Sciences who reached out to most venues to facilitate the launch of the multiple Telemedicine hubs.

The atmosphere around the project was of inspiration and emotional engagement by all those who were involved as they began to feel the impact of the increasing number of calls and visitors to the project. The emotions of the beneficiaries of the service motivated the doctors and the logistic support providers as they began to see the benefit of the new Telemedicine service becoming apparent.

Picture Caption
Online Training by Dr Suhail Chughtai with the help of local teams at various Universities and Medical Institutions with Governor of Punjab reaching out too at some to inaugurate the peripheral Telemedicine Hubs.

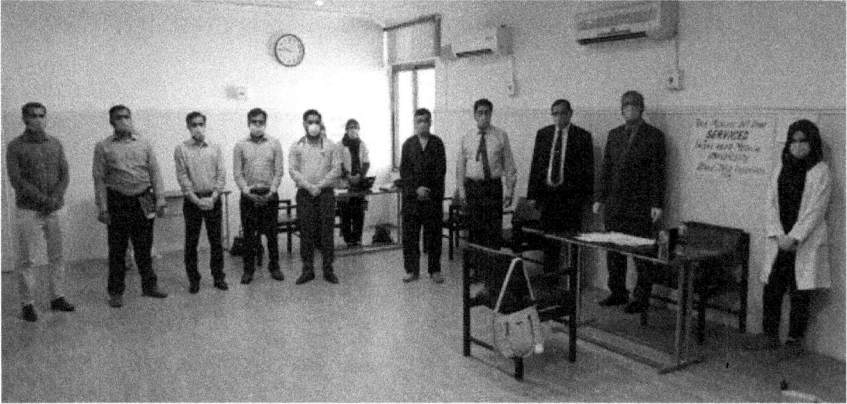

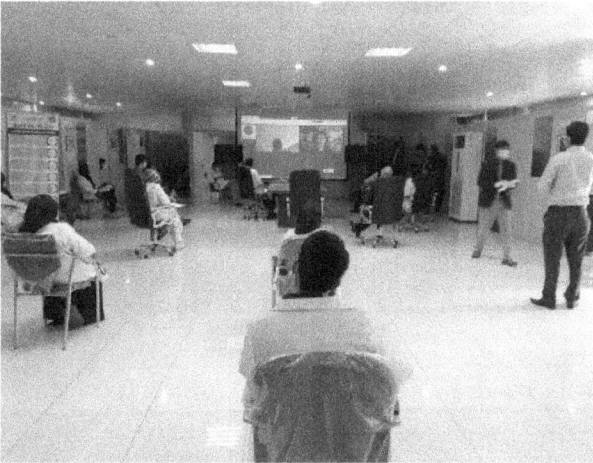

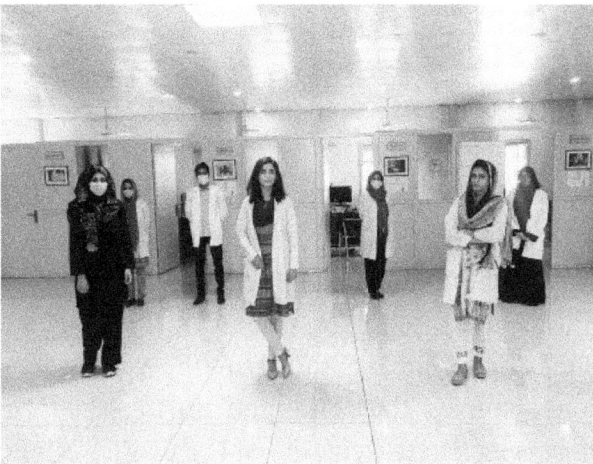

Briefing to the President of Pakistan, Dr Arif Alvi in the first week of April 2020

The President's visit at the site of Primary Telemedicine Hub at the University of Health Sciences, Lahore meant a lot to the project and His Excellency was briefed on the progress made. Dr Alvi expressed personal interest in the field of Telemedicine and felt pleased with the progress made at that stage.

Raising Public Awareness about the Service

To take the service to all members of the public, it was necessary to deploy a marketing strategy to raise awareness of the availability of free medical advice through online consultation. The Governor of Punjab adequately provided this support through his regular tweets along with special advertisements and media reports about the service.

Several media personalities supported the project by recording messages of support such as Reema Khan, Humayun Saeed, Tauqir Nasir and others from the TV and Film industry.

Emerging Stories out of the Telemedicine Helpline

The seed of change were sown at the Press Conference on 12th March 2020, where the shared idea of a new Telemedicine Helpline achieved due attention from the relevant authorities who responded in time and with due ownership. The progress and growth were nurtured by inspirational stories that emerged during the process of providing services to the visitors of the COVID Telemedicine Helpline.

There were instances where people from various countries who sought help through the online doctors of the Telemedicine helpline, mentioned the usefulness of the service that was not available in their own countries. Most of such callers were overseas Pakistanis who had heard about the service on social media or friends and relatives, with some callers from India, the neighbouring country, who were warmly received and provided with free medical advice. Overall, the beneficiaries apart from Pakistan accessed our Telemedicine service from 17 other countries including UAE, Saudi Arabia, Kuwait, Qatar, England, USA and more.

We remain eternally grateful to the young doctors who worked without any salary or financial support providing cover all night long and during the days with dedication and a national spirit to help their country at the critical moment. The public responded with warmth as they felt the benefit and praise started flowing in through the media. A sense of national unity with the health care providers of the Telemedicine helpline started to build up, which encourage the involved young doctors to sustain their energy and enthusiasm.

Chapter Four

Telemedicine Helpline - Scope and Objectives

A Snapshot of the Project's Targets

Author: Dr Suhail Chughtai

The Concept

The Punjab Government deployed "Social Distancing" as a policy to limit the Corona epidemic in March 2020. The essential service of Patient-Doctor physical visits posed a high risk of spreading the Corona epidemic, a challenge which was addressed by setting up the Telemedicine website and appropriate mobile Apps.

Following the Press Briefing on 12th March 2020 in Lahore, I re-designed one of my existing Telemedicine platforms to meet the requirements of a Telemedicine Hotline Service. This re-purposed website, *www.Doctors247. Online* was launched on 19th March 2020 at the University of Health Sciences under the supervision of its Vice Chancellor Prof Dr Javed Akram and inaugurated by the Governor of Punjab, Chaudhary Muhammad Sarwar.

Since COVID-19 forced people to stay at home to mitigate the spread of the virus, Telehealth practices have rapidly expanded. Health care professionals believe that Telehealth will stay even after the end of the pandemic. What was once considered as an experimental way to deliver health care, Telehealth has now become a mainstream delivery system.

The Targeted Impact of www.Doctors247.online on Public Health

- **To reduce crowding at Government Hospitals and Private Clinics**

The influx of patients and their attendants was expected to show a sharp spike which had to be controlled to prevent the rapid spread of COVID-19 epidemic.

To reduce the Mortality and Morbidity of the pandemic affected public

Telehealth has been reported to substantially reduce mortality, reduce the need for admissions to hospital, lower the number of bed days spent in hospital and reduce the time spent in emergency departments of both Government and private medical facilities.

Medical research has demonstrated that, if used correctly, Telehealth can deliver a 15% reduction in emergency room visits; a 20% reduction in emergency admissions; a 14% reduction in elective admissions; a 14% reduction in bed days; and an 8% reduction in tariff costs. More strikingly, the findings showed a 45% reduction in mortality rates.

- **To increase the safety of the Healthcare Professionals**

Doctors, nurses and other healthcare workers are exposed to COVID-19 more than the general public which resulted in a significant number becoming cross - infected with COVID-19 and resulting in an alarming proportion of healthcare staff deaths.

Telemedicine based virtual teleconsultation enables medical advice to be provided without the need for a physical meeting between doctor and patient, thus protecting both of them from the risk of getting or catching infection.

- **To evaluate the Disease penetration in the community**
  The Corona Score Form, embedded in Doctors 247 Online, was an obligatory requirement to be filled in by the doctor during the live teleconsultation. The data entered was designed to be easily extractable and available for review to study the disease burden and demographic distribution.

- **To reduce anxiety of people during home-confined period**
  Being able to meet a doctor in a live audio/video enabled call has been found to be more satisfying than just talking to the doctor over a phone line as proven by independent research studies. Allaying anxiety for those who otherwise would have gone out to meet a doctor in person was one of the objectives aimed for by the virtual teleconsultation through Doctors 247 Online.

- **To deal with Medical Conditions other than COVID-19**
  Several common medical ailments other than COVID-19 were encouraged to be dealt over the Live Tele-consultations to keep the patients confined to their home, which would serve to prevent over-crowding of government hospitals and private clinics in line with the government policy of Social Distancing.

- **To educate Patients and Public at large about Telemedicine**
  The COVID-19 epidemic accelerated the process of finding an alternative means of doctor-patient meeting. This project provided an opportunity for the public to unlearn and relearn an alternative method of meeting the doctor when the rising infection puts both of them at risk.

⋀ **Doctors247 Online**
Powered by Medical City Online, UK

Governor & CM Punjab
Corona Telemedicine Helpline

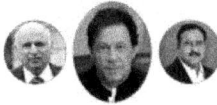

Login as Corona Advisor
لاگ ان اے آئی Connect for Advice
Register as Corona Advisor
Hotline No: 0304 111 2101

Corona Infection Advisors   Partner Institutions   Medical Advisors   Feedback   Covid 19 Info   Software FAQs   Gallery   About us   Contact us

Our Corona Virus Infection Advisors
Tele-consult our Corona Virus Epidemic Advisors to take advice

Search   🔍 ⟳

Telemedicine
Helpline for
CORONA

University of Health
Sciences Lahore

Dr. 01 UHS, Lahore

Telemedicine
Helpline for
CORONA

King Edward
Medical University

Dr. 02 KEMU, Lahore

Telemedicine
Helpline for
CORONA

Shaheed Zulfiqar Ali
Bhutto Medical
University Islamabad

Dr. 03 SZABMU, Islmbad

Telemedicine
Helpline for
CORONA

Nishtar Medical
University Multan

Dr. 04 NMU, Multan

Free Medical Advice on suspected Corona symptoms below:

Visit www.Doctors247.online (website above)
Call 0304 111 2101
Download Android app shown below

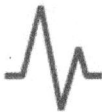

⋀ **Doctors247 Online**
1.8 for Android

Webmaster TVapex

Download APK (21.7 MB)   Versions

- **To empower the Medical Fraternity about Telemedicine**
  The future evolution of healthcare services in Pakistan in order to equalise the physician density through Telemedicine was able to be progressed through this project since doctors would feel more acquainted with the application and more convinced by the usefulness of Telemedicine once they have learnt it under these urgent circumstances.

- **To save costs to the Government for an alternative healthcare delivery pathway**
  Setting up Telemedicine Hubs and connecting to patients via a website is less costly than setting up a conventional physical outpatient clinic. Patients visiting Doctors 24/7 Online website would meet a doctor for a Teleconsultation free of cost and free of transport costs which was both convenient and economical for the patients.

- **To lower the disease burden on patients**
  The Telemedicine helpline served around the clock providing free of charge medical advice in order to ease several burdens on all the patients, especially during the stressful times of the COVID-19 pandemic;

  - The Logistic burden (Travelling to/from clinic)
  - The Social burden (Engaging relatives in the arrangement to go to clinic)
  - The Financial burden (the cost of travelling and doctor's fee)
  - The Emotional burden (being left stranded without medical advice during the lockdown period)

References:

COVID-19 Social Distancing Is Normalizing Telehealth

https://www.govtech.com/health/COVID-19-Social-Distancing-is-Normalizing-Telehealth.html

Impact of Telemedicine on Mortality, Length of Stay and Cost Among Patients in Progressive Care Units: Experience From a Large Healthcare System

https://www.ncbi.nlm.nih.gov/pmc/articles/PMC5908255/

Telemedicine with clinical decision support for critical care: a systematic review

https://pubmed.ncbi.nlm.nih.gov/27756376/

Telehealth can reduce deaths by 45%, study shows

https://www.computerworld.com/article/2500026/telehealth-can-reduce-deaths-by-45---study-shows.html#:~:text=%22The%20first%20set%20of%20initial,Department%20saidn%20in%20a%20statement.

3,635 healthcare workers have tested positive for the coronavirus since the outbreak began, and 35 of those doctors, nurses and health staff did not survive

https://www.aljazeera.com/indepth/features/pakistan-hospitals-struggle-coronavirus-cases-explode-200612084123797.html

Chapter Five

An Introduction to Telemedicine

What, Why and How for Patients, Doctors & Healthcare Administrators

Author: Dr Suhail Chughtai

Author: Dr Suhail Chughtai

Definition and Introduction

Telemedicine is "the process of delivering healthcare services over one or multiple channels of Telecommunication connecting a healthcare provider (a doctor, therapist or nurse) with a patient without a physical meeting." In short, it is the process of a Virtual Medical Consultation over the Internet with a care receiver and a caregiver at two different physical locations.

Essential Elements of a Live Teleconsultation

The basic elements of any Live Medical Teleconsultation can be summed as below, although with increasing level of sophistication, further layers are added:

- A history Taking Interface
- A visual Medical Examination Window
- Medical Notes and Investigation Folders
- A Clinical Decision Portal
- With, at the conclusion, an Auto-summary of the
    Patient-Clinician Encounter

The History Taking Interface

A very valuable part of the patient-clinician interaction is the medical history-taking where the experienced clinician thoroughly assesses the various symptoms of the patient to formulate a diagnosis. The process of taking the medical history involves asking questions about the present complaint, establishing its description, exploring relevant the past medical history of illnesses and surgical operations, the current medications the patient is taking, and other relevant critical individual information.

The Visual Medical Examination Window

For common day-to-day medical practices, many conditions have nothing to show except for pain and discomfort. Other issues may present as a manifestation on the patient's visible skin and mucosa or several physically apparent findings such as muscle wasting, bony deformities, swelling of body parts, etc.

Several common medical conditions can be more closely examined by asking the patient to upload images before their appointment or by instantly using a mobile phone camera during the Teleconsultation. The relevant lesion such as a painful mole, a skin rash or pigmentation, swelling or deformity of a limb can be shown to the examining doctor over live web cam, which helps to reach a differential diagnosis.

Visual examination can safely substitute for most of the physical examination requirements for several specialities, particularly in Psychiatry and Dermatology. With experience, a tactfully conducted visual examination can replace a physical examination to gain sufficient information for reaching a clinical opinion or differential diagnosis.

In specialities like Orthopaedics and Rheumatology, the joint movements can be checked visually to get an impression of the range of motion.

The gap of information can be filled in by patients providing self-checked blood pressure, temperature, and blood glucose readings. A large number of smart gadgets are now available for patients to use at home or through a Practice Assistant at a Telemedicine Spoke to provide additional medical information such as heart and lung sounds, live ECG and even live ultrasound scanning, as well as high-definition imaging of skin, ear, nose and throat or inside the eye.

Medical Notes and Investigation Folders

Advanced scientific developments have resulted in a high degree of accuracy available for medical investigations like MRI scans, nerve conduction studies and echocardiogram, etc., some now benefitting from Artificial Intelligence (AI). These investigations are non-invasive, and they assist in diagnosing medical conditions to confirm or rule out the findings of clinical examination.

The evolving trends in the medical investigation sector have forced several classifications of injuries taught in medical schools to be abolished as they presented no additional value to the diagnosis.

One such example is Pott's classification for ankle fractures which is no longer applicable due to the presence of X-ray facilities. The evolving medico-legal industry has also influenced clinical decision-making as most surgeons would require objective confirmation of physical findings before deciding to operate. One such example is operating for Anterior Cruciate Ligament (ACL) damage (a common sports knee injury) where it is now mandatory to have an MRI scan before operating as reliance on physical examination findings alone for deciding to operate can no longer be defended medico-legally if the surgeon's diagnosis proves to be wrong.

A Clinical Decision Portal

After taking the medical history, the clinician should review the medical notes and investigations followed by the carrying out of a visual medical examination. Then further tests might need to be ordered, or a prescription provided for the patient. In some cases, referral to another relevant medical colleague may be necessary, a facility which an efficient Telemedicine system should be designed to provide.

The dispatch of medical investigation requests or e-prescriptions can be set up to be provided automatically for intended providers.

An Auto-summary of the Patient-Clinician Encounter

Telemedicine software should have this embedded feature integrated using AI for various elements of the observations and comments recorded by the clinician during or after the consultation, creating an auto-summary of the patient-clinician encounter.

Such an auto-summary of the Teleconsultation should then be kept as a record of the patient-clinician encounter for future reference.

An efficient Telemedicine System for General Teleconsultation

The above elements complete the anatomy of a basic Telemedicine system, as long as they are embedded in a single and secure interface, the idea of providing remote medical care can be well served. The five pillars, therefore, are summed up again:

- A History Taking Interface
- A Visual Medical Examination Window
- Medical Notes and Investigation Folders
- A Clinical Decision Portal
- An auto-summary of the Patient-Clinician Encounter

Difference between Telehealth, Telemedicine and Telecare

What is Telehealth?

The Telecare Services Association defines Telehealth as the "Delivery of Healthcare Services remotely through Telecommunications Technology". Telehealth is defined as "the transmission of data of patients (documents, images, audio, video, etc.) between separate physical locations to diagnose and monitor suitable medical conditions remotely". The term is used synonymously for a range of portals working together to facilitate healthcare, promote public health and deliver health education via Telecommunications Technologies.

What is Telemedicine?

Telemedicine is "the process of delivering healthcare services over one or multiple channels of Telecommunication connecting a healthcare provider (a doctor, therapist or nurse) with a patient without a physical meeting". In short, it is the process of carrying out a Virtual Medical Consultation over the Internet with the care receiver and the caregiver at two different physical locations.

What is Telecare?

Telecare is defined as providing healthcare services via remote monitoring utilising equipment, gadgets and Telecommunication technology". Remote monitoring via modern or smart medical gadgets to record BP, Pulse, Blood Glucose, single-lead ECG, etc., can be carried out using a connected healthcare system. The documented findings are interpreted during Virtual or Physical Consultations. Telecare can be a standalone service, or it can be part of a Telemedicine portal.

Structural types of Telemedicine

Live or Synchronous Telemedicine occurs when the patient and healthcare provider are interacting in real-time. In the past, this was typically a telephone conversation between the care staff and the patient. This is now gradually being replaced with the use of a live two-way audio-video interface created with appropriate Telemedicine Software.

Store & Forward or Asynchronous Telemedicine occurs when the patient's health information is forwarded electronically and stored for review by the relevant healthcare provider at a subsequent time, who then sends medical advice back to the patient. The steps of the process are mostly carried out offline, not in real-time.

A Hybrid of the above two types implies conversion from one to another such as an asynchronous consultation needing a live video consultation necessitated by the results of an investigation such as an MRI scan or a Tissue Biopsy that requires urgent action and counselling for the patient

Functional types of Telemedicine

Direct Telemedicine involves a patient having a Teleconsultation directly with the healthcare provider without needing a coordinator or an assistant such as creating an account on a Telemedicine website, searching, and connecting with a doctor or healthcare provider.

Assisted Telemedicine, also known as Hub and Spoke Telemedicine typically involves the assistance of a trained Telemedicine Coordinator who would help the patient to register, connect, and be examined over the Teleconsultation after the patient has visited a Telemedicine facility (Telemedicine Spoke) and is then connected to a remotely based clinician (at the Telemedicine Hub).

Automated Telemedicine or Telecare usually entails a patient using smart medical gadgets for recording vital signs like blood pressure, pulse, ECG, blood glucose and blood oxygen that can be transmitted using Bluetooth enabled mobile devices connected as smart gadgets. Once the mobile devices are connected, it is possible to set up an automated transfer of vital signs readings into the Telemedicine interface for subsequent review at the in-person or virtual appointments with the healthcare provider. Critical value thresholds can be set up such as extremely low blood pressure, low pulse rate or very high blood sugar, etc., that will then trigger alarms at the doctor or nurse's end to ensure prompt intervention takes place. This method is quite popular for the care of the elderly at home, or a post-operative patient discharged home but needing monitoring till fully recovered.

Mobile Health typically involves the use of healthcare Apps on smart-phones or tablets to capture medical data and convey the health information two way within a pre-defined Clinical Decision Support System for managing medical conditions.

Clinical types of Telemedicine

General Telemedicine Service implies an outpatient Teleconsultation interface that fits general history taking and examination for day-to-day common ailments, usually well adapted to the needs of primary care physicians.

Specialised Telemedicine Service would imply a specific flow of the patient history, specifically relevant to a particular speciality assisted by an in-built digital tool kit to meet the needs of the speciality Teleconsultation, e.g., Tele-cardiology, Tele-dermatology, Tele-physiotherapy, Tele-psychiatry etc. Specific digital tools are usually embedded within the Teleconsultation interface with or without connected smart medical gadgets such as a pulse-oximeter, a glucometer, etc., to make Teleconsultation as close to an in-person visit as possible.

Super-specialised Telemedicine Service would imply highly specialised Telemedicine software combining an embedded software toolkit and connected specialised smart gadgets such as a Tele-ultrasound device, digital microscope, or ophthalmoscope etc. This type of highly specialised software can be layered with the relevant interface of artificial intelligence for enhanced functionality to support the accuracy of clinical decision making.

Types of Telemedicine based on Audio-Video Channels

Single Channel Telemedicine Software is where the audio and video channels from within the software controls are not switch-able. So, a camera or microphone attached to the device (computer/smart phone or tablet) are going to be fixed input devices to assist the clinician in medical examination.

Multi-channel Telemedicine Software is where the audio and video channels from within the software controls are switchable. So, a camera or microphone attached to the device (computer/smart phone or tablet) are NOT going to be fixed input devices to assist the clinician in medical examination.

Any other cameras (like Dermascope, ENT Camera, Ultrasound probe etc) or alternative audio input (Cardiac auscultation device, pre-natal Fetoscope) can be switched from within the Software. The benefit of this sophisticated Telemedicine feature is to provide facility to a Coordinator at a Telemedicine Spoke to switch easily with one click between various cameras and audio medical gadgets to facilitate various specialists at the other end of a Hub and Spoke Telemedicine Clinic.

Benefits of Telemedicine

Benefits to Patients

- Telemedicine visits save time as an average time of 2 hours are needed for an in-person visit (combined travel, clinic wait and physician time) compared to 15 minutes (combined waiting and physician time).
- No need to make travel arrangements.
- Confidence and convenience equal to that of a home visit by a doctor.
- Prompt availability of a doctor to match the patient's schedule on a workday, out of hours or even weekends.
- Automated remote monitoring of vital signs and medical conditions are now possible.
- Improved engagement and focus between a patient and a doctor.
- Availability of a doctor outside the geographical region of the patient.
- Formation of a Medical Board (often called a Multi-Disciplinary Clinic in the UK) of different doctors in various locations is now possible in a short time and at less cost.
- Prevention of the risk of cross-infection, both receiving or transmitting infection during the journey to/from the clinic and at the clinic, COVID-19 epidemic being one example, others being seasonal flu and skin infections.
- Teleconsultations are often less costly to the patient, and most certainly where one involves travelling out of a city or country.
- On average, elective Teleconsultations would cost a hospital 30% less than in-person visits.

- Electronic Records can be maintained by uploading files or taking photos of lab reports, X-rays and uploading them to the Patient-dashboard of the Telemedicine software.
- Patient satisfaction is often improved as the doctor is promptly available, and early intervention is possible.
- Better healthcare as early intervention is possible, such as picking up a suspicious skin mole early before the potentially cancerous lesion spreads further.
- A reduced number of hospital visits are needed, thus less loss of work or business commitments.
- Privacy of the Teleconsultation visits a desirable attribute, for instance, when some patients, due to their social position, delay their psychiatric check-up to avoid being seen at the psychiatric clinic waiting room.
- The overall effect on the patient using the service is to lower the logistical, disease, financial and emotional burdens. Several international surveys have indicated that on average, 85% of patients who have used Teleconsultation once would opt for it again.

Benefits to Healthcare Providers (Doctors, Nurses, Therapists)

- Widening of outreach without leaving their physical location thus available to patients far from clinics in the same city, other cities, or even other countries.
- Less building or staffing requirements to widen clinic practice needed for Telemedicine practice, thus less cost required to set up Telemedicine practice.
- More satisfaction to the patient as doctor/healthcare provider being more readily available.

- Improves Clinical work flow while enhancing practice efficiency
- Reduces patient no-shows or failure to attend by more than 50% reported by several independent surveys.
- The prevention of contagious infections such as seasonal flu. Telemedicine has become the preferable means of carrying out a consultation by both patient and doctor duringthe COVID-19 epidemic where a significant number of healthcare professionals lost lives due to catching the virus by providing in-person medical practice.
- Better management of the patient's health records, vital sign values, important clinical findings captured on images taken by the patient
- The overall effect is higher patient satisfaction, enhanced work flow efficiency, increased practice revenue and reduced clinic overhead.

Benefits to the Healthcare System, Institution or Government

Telemedicine can improve the overall standard of care. A national study in the UK indicated that "if correctly used", Telehealth can deliver a 15% reduction in accident and emergency visits, 20% reduction in emergency admissions, 14% reduction in elective admissions, 14% reduction in bed days and an 8% reduction in tariff costs. Another significant finding was a 45% reduction of mortality rates which most likely related to timely intervention and facility of remote monitoring (Gornall, 2012).

Ref: https://www.bmj.com/bmj/section-pdf/187582?path=/bmj/345/7865 Feature.full.pdf
Gornall, J. (2012). Does Telemedicine deserve the green light? BMJ, 345(jul10 1), pp e4622

Telemedicine improves Clinical Governance.
A prominent Australian study reports that Telehealth incorporation into the healthcare delivery service improves clinical governance. Telehealth was noticed as enabling improved quality, integration, and implementation of evidence-based care, and to be significant support for the rural health workforce. Telehealth was reported to be beneficial by reducing adverse events, improving health outcomes, offering an increased patient choice of service delivery, and improving access to services for rural areas and home care.

Ref: https://journals.sagepub.com/doi/abs/10.1258/jtt.2011.110808
Wade, V.A., Eliott, J.A. and Hiller, J.E. (2012). A qualitative study of ethical, medico-legal and clinical governance matters in Australian telehealth services. Journal of Telemedicine and Telecare, 18(2), pp.109–114.

Telemedicine improves Healthcare economy.
Telemedicine adoption improves the cost efficiency of a healthcare system. An exemplar study shows that the use of Telemedicine for retinal screening was beneficial and cost-effective for diabetes management, with an incremental cost-effectiveness ratio between \$113.48/quality-adjusted life year (QALY) and \$3,328.46/QALY (adjusted to 2017 inflation rate). Similarly, the use of telemonitoring and telephone reminders was cost-effective in diabetes management (Lee and Lee, 2018).

Ref: https://www.liebertpub.com/doi/abs/10.1089/dia.2018.0098
Lee, J.Y. and Lee, S.W.H. (2018). Telemedicine Cost–Effectiveness for Diabetes Management: A Systematic Review. Diabetes Technology & Therapeutics, 20(7), pp.492–500.

Telemedicine improves Electronic Medical Records management. Telemedicine adoption has been demonstrated to improve record-keeping when compared with in-person visits.

Telemedicine reduces disease burden in the community. Chronic diseases present a significant demand on the healthcare system of any institution or government due to their demand on outpatient visits, in-patient beds occupancy and load on lab work.

One high profile study has demonstrated that the deployment of Telemedicine for managing "Chronic Heart Failure, Chronic Obstructive Pulmonary Disease and Stroke" reported empirical evidence attesting to the potential of Telemedicine for addressing problems of access to care, quality of care, and healthcare costs in the management of the three chronic diseases chosen for this review (Bashshur et al., 2014).

Ref: https://www.ncbi.nlm.nih.gov/pmc/articles/PMC4148063/
Bashshur, R.L., Shannon, G.W., Smith, B.R., Alverson, D.C., Antoniotti, N., Barsan, W.G., Bashshur, N., Brown, E.M., Coye, M.J., Doarn, C.R., Ferguson, S., Grigsby, J., Krupinski, E.A., Kvedar, J.C., Linkous, J., Merrell, R.C., Nesbitt, T., Poropatich, R., Rheuban, K.S., Sanders, J.H., Watson, A.R., Weinstein, R.S. and Yellowlees, P. (2014). The Empirical Foundations of Telemedicine Interventions for Chronic Disease Management. Telemedicine Journal and e-Health, [online] 20(9), pp.769–800. Available at: https://www.ncbi.nlm.nih.gov/pmc/articles/ PMC4148063/

Telemedicine can facilitate Governments in managing Epidemics in a better way. The use of Telemedicine in epidemic situations has a high potential in improving epidemiological investigations, disease control, and clinical case management.Teleconsultations would help to assess the disease burden, evaluate, and categorise individuals making it feasible for dispatching the necessary help and instructing isolation wherever necessary.

The advantage of using Telemedicine as a tool expands to protecting doctors as well as patients from catching or transmitting an infectious airborne disease pathogen (Ohannessian, 2015).

Ref: https://www.ncbi.nlm.nih.gov/pmc/articles/PMC7148594/

Telemedicine makes it possible for Governments to study disease pattern and modify or create health policies.

The use of Telemedicine in epidemic situations has a high potential for improving epidemiological investigations, disease control, and clinical case management.

Teleconsultations, correctly documented, can facilitate the assessment of the disease burden, evaluate, and categorise individuals making it feasible for dispatching the necessary help and provide rapid isolation instructions wherever necessary.

Benefits to the environment and community

Telemedicine makes Healthcare Greener.

In-person visits have reduced the need for patient transport, paperwork production and transmission and consumption of in-office services by both patients and clinician, which continues to pollute the environment and enlarging the carbon footprint.

By adopting Telemedicine and health information technology, time, energy, raw materials (such as paper and plastic), and fuel consumption needed for travelling can be reduced thus minimising the carbon footprint raised by the healthcare industry (Yellowlees et al., 2010).

Ref: https://www.liebertpub.com/doi/abs/10.1089/tmj.2009.0105

Telemedicine democratises the Healthcare Service for Consumers (Patients). The development of a Telemedicine culture, where a patient is engaged in a better way through live and personalised one-to-one online consultation can result in more patients being given better access to medical care and potentially a better consultation experience.

Telemedicine empowers a patient by sharing the responsibility of care and offers an opportunity to question steps of management during a Teleconsultation.

Telemedicine ready patients are offered an online dashboard to add information periodically such as BP, Blood Glucose readings or uploaded ECGs, radiographic or clinical Images. The wealth of healthcare information about oneself available to a patient is recognised to engage a patient better.

The compliance with a treatment plan has been confirmed to be better where a patient is informed and engaged. Telemedicine democratises a community and overall helps raise the health standard of the public (Tang and Smith, 2016).

Ref: https://jamanetwork.com/journals/jama/article-abstract/2556028. Tang, P.C. and Smith, M.D. (2016). Democratisation of Health Care. JAMA, 316(16), p.1663.

Chapter Six

Power of the Software Design of Doctors 24/7 Telemedicine Helpline

Simplified to Bits Yet a Clinically Powerful Online Portal

Author: Dr Suhail Chughtai

Considering the limitations faced in terms of the short time for training doctors and the lack of familiarity of Telemedicine services by the general public, it was essential to keep the Telemedicine interface user friendly to both doctors and patients alike, yet fully functional for a meaningful healthcare-related encounter over the internet.

Patient registration and login – Connection with a Doctor within 60 seconds

- The patient with suspected COVID-19 symptoms would visit the website using a desktop computer, a laptop, a smartphone, or a tablet. An android doctors247.online mobile app is also available from the Google Play Store.
- The available doctors from various Telemedicine hubs were connected to the website and are shown as *Blinking Icons*.
- The patient can click on any of the *Blinking Icons* and reach the doctor by providing their name, mobile phone number and city.
- The Online doctor will then get a beep sound as soon a visitor hits the waiting room, the doctor then hits their Go Live" button at his or her end to indicate they are in the office and ready to receive the patient.

- The visitor's device will ring and show a clear button on the screen, asking him or her to then connect to the doctor.
- Both doctor and patient immediately meet in the virtual live video consultation room where the doctor will take the patient through the Corona scoring form or go through a routine primary medical consultation if their call was medical but not about a Corona infection.
- During the virtual consultation, a routine history-taking and visual examination are carried out.
- The doctor will advise the patient on the next steps, based upon the Corona-Form score and the findings on visual examination.
- The patient has access to upload any medical lab results they have available during the live Teleconsultation to assist the doctor further in their medical assessment.
- The doctor was provided with diagrams and images to the patient on how to take the necessary precautions for social distancing and social isolation if applicable.
- The doctor was provided with a facility to prescribe medications online if required and to request certain medical investigations if necessary.
- Once seen, any patient once seen can re-visit the service for a follow-up Teleconsultation using their mobile number as their user-name.
- The record of any previous Teleconsultation or e-prescriptions are kept in the patient's electronic dashboard for both follow-up appointments and for governance purposes.

The Home or the Landing page showing blinking tabs of the available online doctors. The offline doctors do not blink

After clicking on one of the online doctors's tab, the following screen appears asking for basic information to be filled in which usually takes 30 seconds or so to complete.

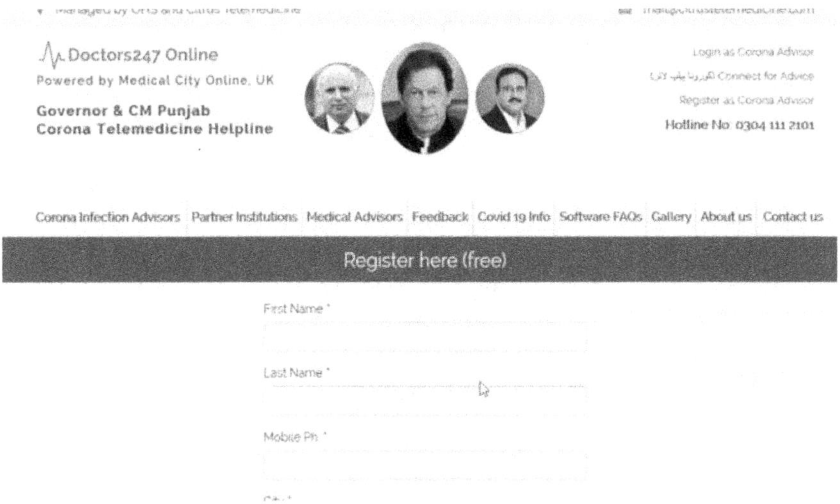

Then by hitting the "Connect" button the patient will land in the doctor's virtual waiting room and the doctor is notified on-screen by a blinking button "1 patient waiting" and a beep sound on his computer terminal.

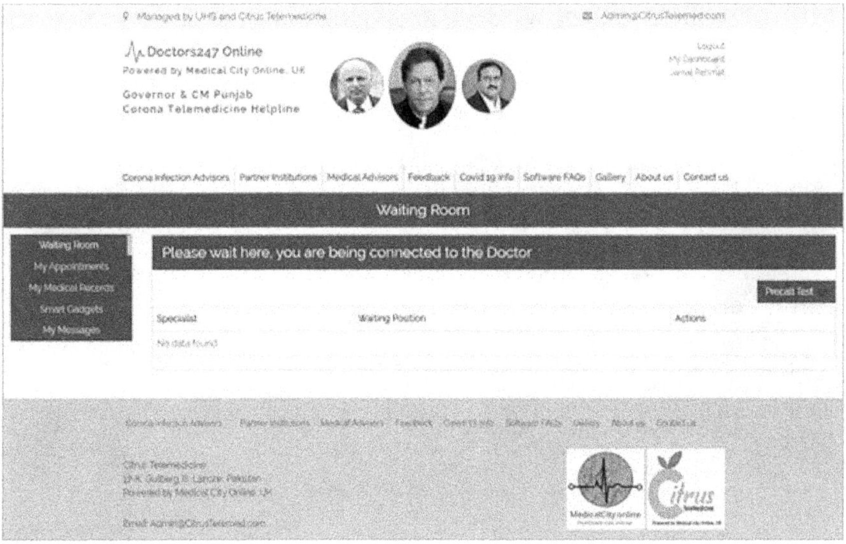

The following few screen-shots have been taken at the "Doctor's end" to show how the process of free medical advice is completed, with the visitor or patient taken through step by step. The doctor is shown in a small inset (top right), while the patient's image is in the larger image in the centre of the window at the start of the Teleconsultation.

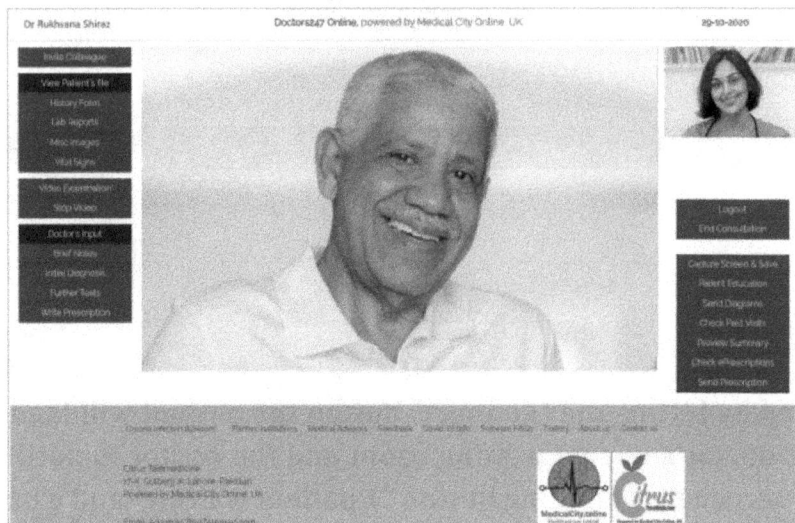

Here, the doctor (top inset window) is taking the patient (bottom inset window) through the Corona Scoring Form and is filling information while the patient is also able to see the form at their end at the same time.

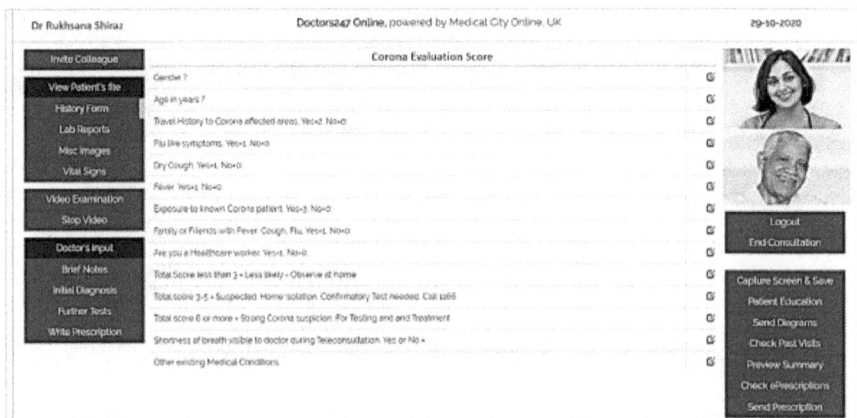

Here the doctor is looking at a Lab Result which the visiting patient can share easily by taking a picture of the report and uploading it through their side screen using clearly marked buttons.

Here the doctor is looking at an X-rays film which the visiting patient can share easily by taking a picture of their x-ray film and by uploading it through their side screen using clearly marked buttons.

This screenshot shows the doctor asking questions about simple parameters which some patients have already recorded at home such as body temperature, pulse, blood pressure, blood glucose (Diabetics using their own home glucometer) or oxygen saturation (where people have bought devices for home care as the often do in Pakistan).

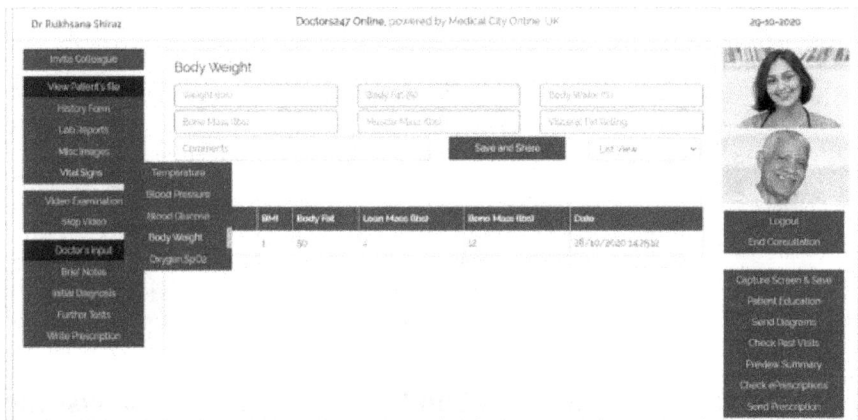

This screen shows the doctor using their Video Examination button to carry out a Visual Examination or and asking more questions as a "face-to-face" virtual consultation.

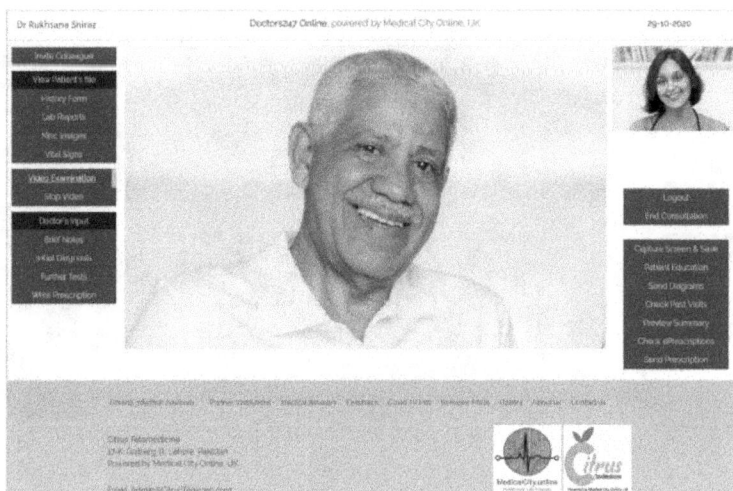

At this point, the doctor is now able to type brief notes to document a summary of their clinical impression, which shall be used to build up the "Electronic Medical Record" of this Teleconsultation.

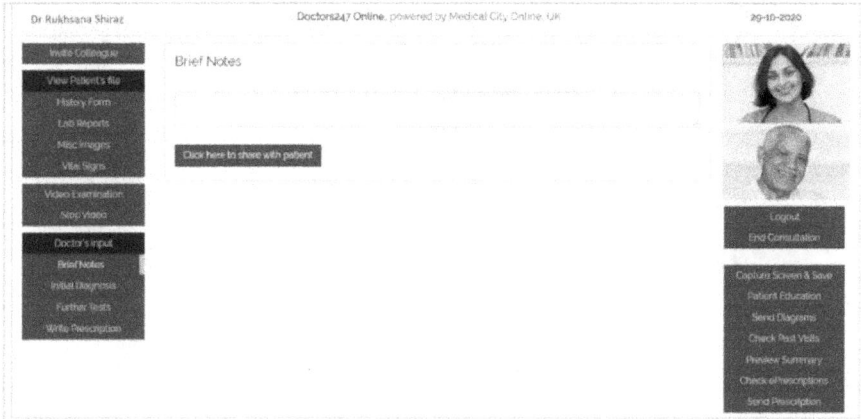

Now the doctor is inserting a "Provisional Diagnosis" based upon the "history of illness", "review of medical test results", "knowledge of vital sign readings" and "impression made on the Visual Examination".

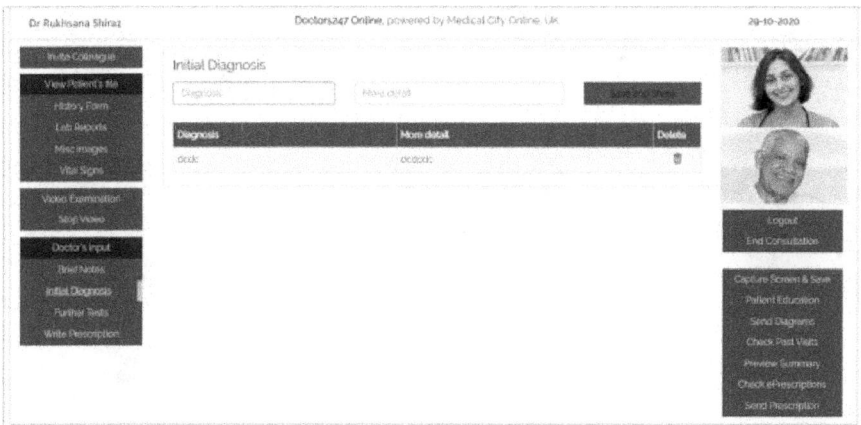

At this point, the doctor can suggest to the patient to have further tests such as Complete Blood Count, Liver Function Tests, Chest X-rays.

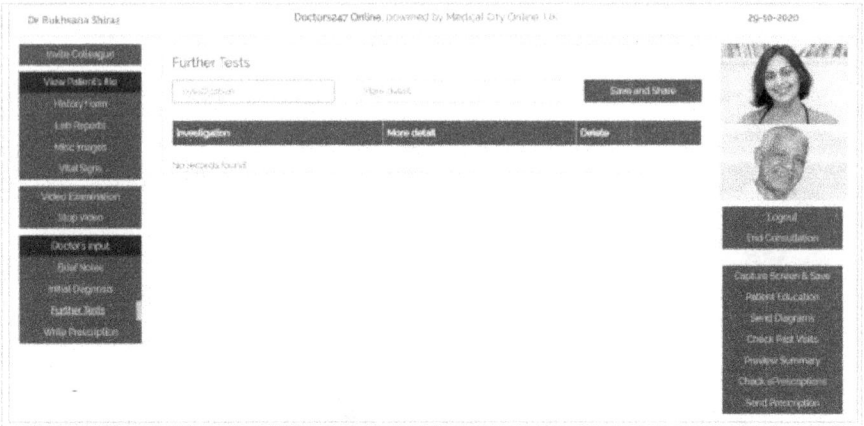

The doctor may now write a prescription which shall not only become part of the electronic medical record of this Teleconsultation but is also be downloadable at the patient's end in order to obtain it from the pharmacist.

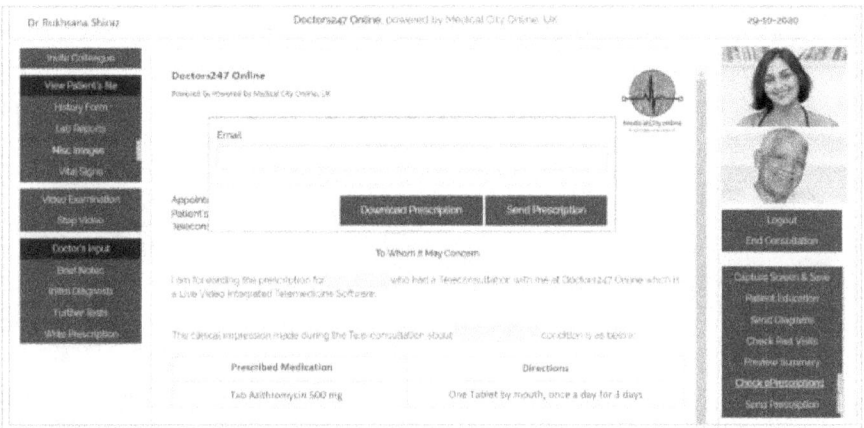

During the Teleconsultation, the Doctors 24/7 Online Telemedicine Software provides a facility for the doctor to capture and save within the patient's record any visual clinical findings such as 'COVID fingers and toes' Skin Rashes, etc., not only record-keeping but also for a visual comparison at the follow-up examination.

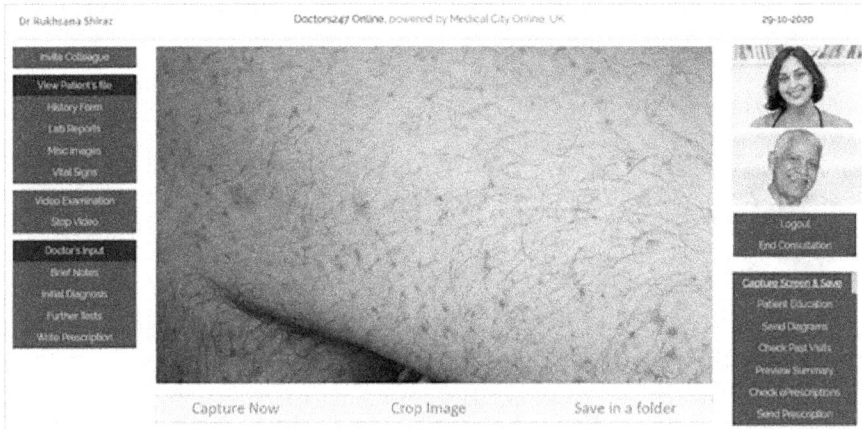

Additionally, the doctor can share YouTube videos with the patient to demonstrate procedures such as handwashing technique explained by a COVID Medical Expert (Dr Somia Iqtadar) as exemplified in this screen-shot. The patients while watching can ask questions to clarify any points during the short clips.

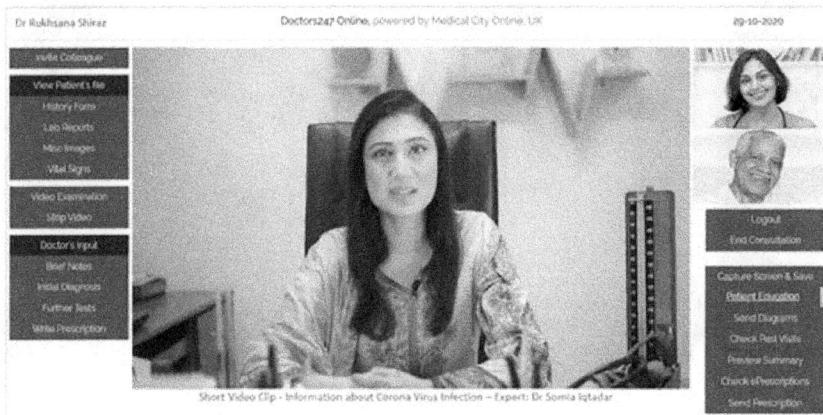

This screen shows the doctor sharing a series of Pakistan educational images in Urdu and answering any questions that a patient may have while being educated on preventive measures.

During the consultation the doctor can send any images requested by the patient via the email address of the patient. The Download Diagram button is also shown at the patient end who can then save it on his/her device for viewing later.

For a follow-up Teleconsultation, the doctor is able to check all the past visits to review each previous Teleconsultation's summary saved within the software system.

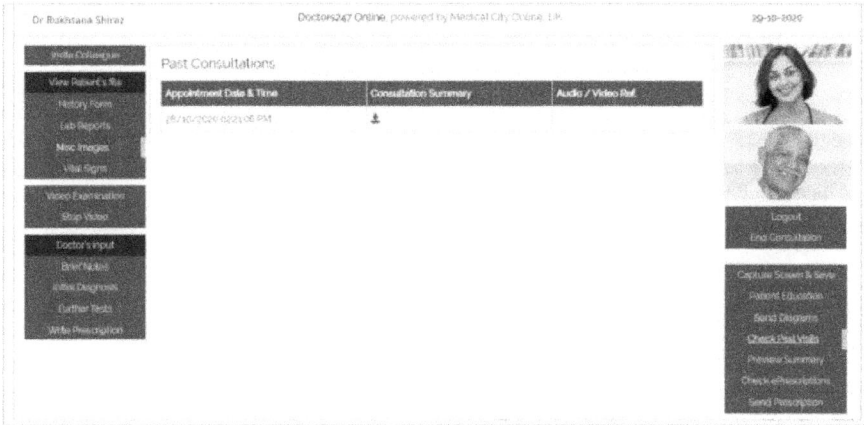

Before finishing, the doctor has an option to review the Summary of this Teleconsultation which has been built up automatically (using Artificial intelligence or AI) using the information registered by the doctor during this virtual encounter.

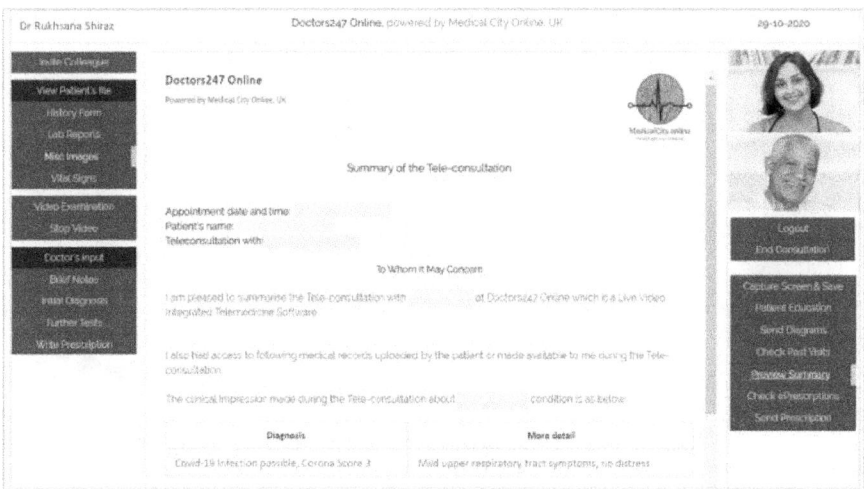

In the same way, the doctor can now review any prescription they have provided and explain any points if necessary. A doctor mentioning specific points about taking medication with the prescription in front of the patient screen will add to the confidence of the patient.

Finally, before finishing, the prescription can be downloaded at the patient end on their device for taking it manually to the chemist or the doctor is able to send it directly to the central office of the Pharmacy chain who will then arrange a dispatch of medications to the patient's home if requested.

Summary of the Software Design

I re-designed my generic Telemedicine Software while attempting to keep the bare minimum features to lighten up the load on bandwidth, to ease the learning curve, yet deliver the intended outcome. Here I share a summary of the features of Doctors 24/7 Online to serve as the Corona Telemedicine Helpline Interface.

Scope

Doctors 24/7 Online was purposed to assist the patient-doctor consultation from a distance using Live Audio-Video Technology seamlessly embedded within a clinical decision support system made up of an electronic medical records portal, an instant appointment system, a prescription interface, an investigation request portal, a patient education library of images and short videos along with an image capture facility. This design would also serve the following types of Telemedicine service:

- Direct Telemedicine service: A patient to doctor contact without any facilitator
- Assisted Telemedicine service: Using a Tele-coordinator managed Spoke connecting a patient to a doctor at a Telemedicine Hub

Features of Doctors 24/7 Online Telemedicine Software

Medical City Online provided a professionally enriched and seamlessly unified Clinical Telemedicine System, much more than just a video conferencing interface. The following additional features were provided through this software:

1. An Instant Appointment System

- Instant connectivity to free medical advice within 30-60 seconds from the point a patient clicks on the blinking tab of the online doctor

2. A Practice Management System

- Patient Registration using basic parameters
- Setting up doctor's individual logins
- Placing Doctors under certain groups such as a Medical University tab, etc
- Doctor to turn on and turn off his/her waiting room during short breaks
- Patient to arrive in a digital waiting room of the doctor clicked by the patient with due notifications at both ends

3. A Basic Electronic Medical Record for the patients

- Patient uploading an image from a computer or smartphone
- Patient capturing and uploading an image using a webcam or smartphone camera
- Doctor capturing important clinical findings or records using the patient's webcam or smartphone camera and
- saving it to the patient's record
- All notes made during the Teleconsultation saved within appropriate folders

4. A Manual Entry of Vital Signs readings

- Arterial Pulse, Blood Pressure, Body Temperature
- Blood Glucose (Glucometer entry), Pulse Oximeter readings

5. **A Live Teleconsultation in HD Video (with the patient and Doctor in real-time in two windows)**

- The Doctor and Patient can view Medical Records simultaneously
- The Doctor should have large video display area to facilitate visual examination
- The Doctor is provided with a drawing tool to draw on images or test results to help explain details of the consultation

6. **An Electronic Waiting Room for doctor's patients (Digital Queueing Protocol)**

- With a digital Waiting Room queue system with three patient room
- With the Doctor having the ability to send sound and screen notification to the next patient

7. **Providing Clinical Audit and Clinical Practice Guidelines**

- Includes a facility for adding forms for Disease Scoring or special condtion-based forms to assist information collection and setting up medical practice guidelines
- Facilitates exporting data in easy steps for Audit, Research and Disease Burden review

8. **Facilitating Clinical and Management Governance**

- Designed to export Clinical and Demographic information for Key Performance Indices for Healthcare providers involved in the service.
- Providing compliance with the healthcare providers and designed to facilitate data export

- Including Patient-Doctor encounter notes available for later performance review

9. Providing Patient Education Modules

- Providing a facility to pre-loaded images for patient education
- Including short, embedded video clips viewable without leaving the Live Teleconsultation interface so that any patient's questions can be answered immediately

10. Including Integrated with support services

- Pharmacy – With the potential for Home delivery or collection
- Pathology Lab – With the option for a Home venepuncture service or booking a visit Home drawing of blood sample or visit to the lab
- Radiology Lab – With the option for booking an appointment to the nearest Radiology lab

11. An e-Prescription download availability

- The Patient can download or choose to have it emailed to him/her
- The Prescription becomes part of the EMR/Consultation

12. Providing an Auto-summary and Voice-to-Text Transcription built- in

- The Doctor's notes saved as an Auto-Summary
- An Auto-summary is available to the patient as a downloadable pdf document
- The Teleconsultation can provide summaries of past visits available at a follow-up visit

13. A Choice of Devices

- At the Doctor end: Laptop, Desktop PC (Windows/Apple)
- At the Patient end: Laptop, Desktop PC (Windows/Apple), Smart Phones, Tablets
- At facility to provide Website Mobile Responsiveness – 100%
- Flexibility of Mobile Apps – iOS (App Store) and Android (Google Store)

Healthcare Data Security standards met by Doctors 24/7 Online

Quality Compliance and Security of Hardware Server Base

The Telemedicine Software has met the challenge of securing healthcare information put into the hands of clinicians, health and care professionals, and the general public. The HSCN (the Health and Social Care Network) ensures that health and social care unite to transform patient care. HSCN connectivity supports the digital transformation of the world's top healthcare systems, like NHS Hospital systems in the UK.

We host healthcare data at an approved HSCN Consumer Network-Service Provider (CN-SP), providing secure cloud services with connectivity to both the Internet and HSCN. The healthcare data used by our Telemedicine Software is based at a secure, certified cloud hosting service.

We are GDPR compliant and meet the standards of the NHS Data Security and Protection (DSP) toolkit.

The healthcare data hosted and stored at Medical City Online Telemedicine Software Cloud Server meets the following stringent requirements:

- Managed Hosting with HSCN Connectivity
- Protective Monitoring compliant with NCSC GPG-13
- SC cleared administrators & data centre team
- ISO 27001 physical data centre security
- ISO Certification 22301 – Approved Business Continuity Management System
- ISO Certification 9001 – Complies to internal Quality Management System (QMS)
- ISO Certification 14001 – Complies to Carbon Footprint Environmental Standards
- PCI Compliance – For additional financial transactional security
- NICEIC Electrical Contractor – Accreditation for high quality of electrical work to minimize shut down or downtime due to electrical failure
- New HSCN Connections and N3 transition
- Hosting existing HMG accredited services, including PASF
- PAS 2060 – Certified as 100% carbon neutral
- Cyber Essentials – Compliance to International Data Security Compliance for cyberattacks
- Cloud Framework – Compliant to International standards of G-Cloud 11 Framework

Our International Standards of PHI security

Our Telemedicine Software Data Management is compliant with international standards of "Patient Health Information" (PHI) General Data Protection Regulation (GDPR) requirements.

- Encryption of all personal information, e.g., user-name, first & last name, email, phone number etc.
- Encryption of all user password with a hash algorithm to prevent password decryption
- Encryption of all patient uploaded documents such as Lab reports, Medical records, photos etc.
- Encryption of Query String ID in the URL
- Incorporation of Anti-forgery Token for CSRF in NET
- Incorporation of a Parameterized Stored Procedure and Entity for the prevention of SQL Injection
- Inclusion of Audio-Video Communication between doctor and patient compliant with international standards such as Health Insurance Portability & Accountability (HIPAA)
- Registration with the Data Protection Act of International Standards – (ICO, UK)
- Domain Security – with Secure Socket Layer certification

Our Platform / Architecture

- Backend Database Association with SQL Server 2016

Our Web App - Application Development Platform

- Asp.Net MVC In C# language

Our Application Hosting

- Windows dedicated server hosting from UKFAST, Manchester

Our Minimum Service Logistic Specifications

- PC or Mac (Laptop or Desktop) with minimum i3 processor (i5 recommended)
- Operating system Windows 10 or Mac OS
- 2 GB RAM (4 GB recommended) and 10 GB HDD
- Internet speed requirement is 500 KB/sec (1.0 GB recommended) available at the device unshared
- HD Webcam, noise-cancelling microphone, speaker

Smartphones and Tablets released in the market after 2017 January onwards

Browser compatibility and Mobile Responsiveness is compatible with
Google Chrome, Firefox Mozilla, Apple Safari, Opera

Official Recognition of Medical City Online Telemedicine Software

Medical City Online Telemedicine Software has received National recognition by the Government of Punjab and approved by several Medical Universities. The local team on the ground was Citrus Telemedicine, an SECP approved company in Pakistan.

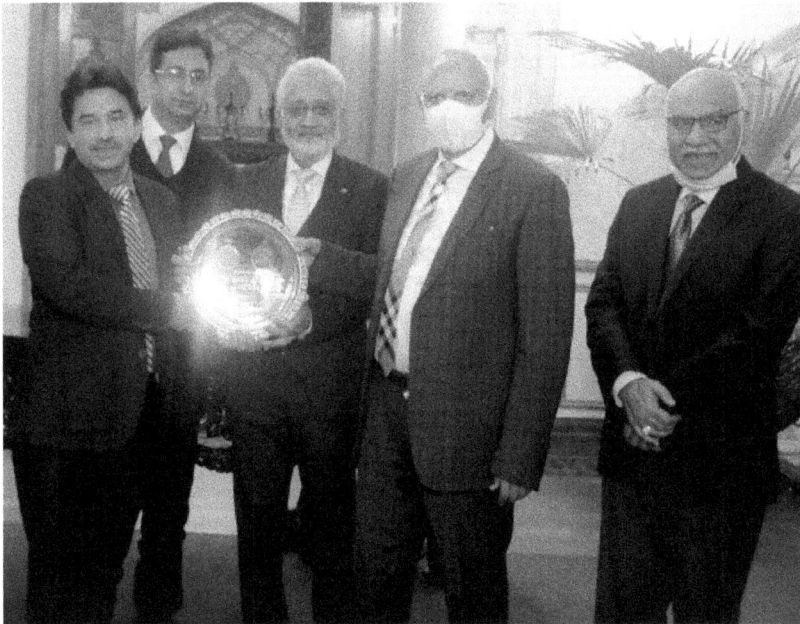

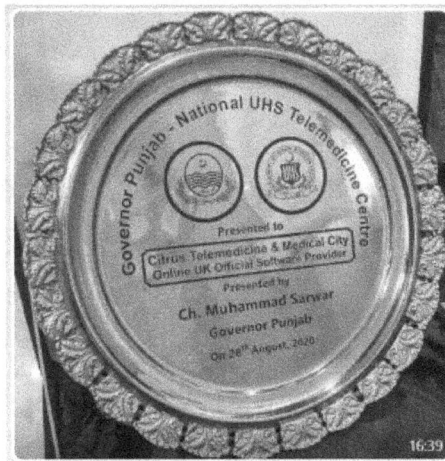

Chapter Seven

COVID-19 in Pakistan

An Overview of the Menace of the Disease & How it was handled in Pakistan

Author: Dr Somia Iqtadar

COVID-19 Virus, an overview
The Infectious nature of COVID-19
Common symptoms of COVID-19 infection
Clinical Classification of Disease
Vaccine for COVID 19
Telemedicine and COVID-19

What is an Epidemic?

An epidemic is an outbreak of a disease that spreads quickly and affects many people at the same time. An outbreak occurs when there is a sudden increase in the number of cases of a disease. It generally describes an increase that was not anticipated. An outbreak can occur in a community, geographical area, or several countries, and during this, the disease is actively spreading.

Examples of past epidemics are the 1918 Spanish flu epidemic, the measles outbreak from 1981 to 1991, and the whooping cough epidemic in 2014 with 9,935 cases reported in California, USA.

A pandemic is a type of epidemic that relates to geographic spread and describes a disease that affects an entire country or the whole world.

An epidemic becomes a pandemic when it spreads over significant geographical areas and affects a large percentage of the population. In short, a pandemic is an epidemic on a national or global level. A pandemic describes an infectious disease where we see significant and ongoing person-to-person spread in multiple countries around the world at the same time. It's often caused by a new virus or a new strain of virus that has not circulated within people for a long time. Being novel, humans have little to no immunity against the virus, and it spreads quickly causing more deaths. Owing to its vast impact, it creates social disruption and economic loss.

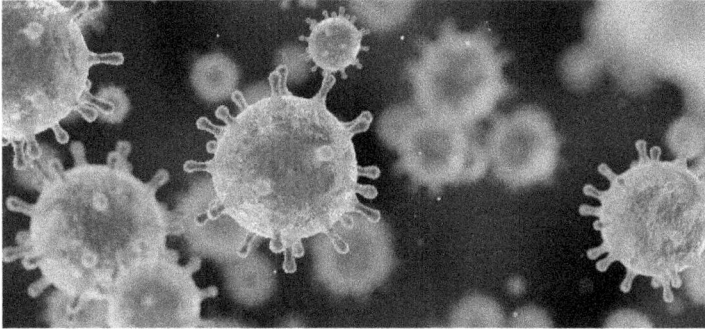

The last time a pandemic occurred was in 2009 with swine flu, which experts think killed hundreds of thousands of people. Other examples of past pandemics are the flu pandemic of 1968, the HIV/AIDS pandemic from the early 1980's peaking in 1997, and the Bubonic plague in the 14th Century.

A pandemic is different from an epidemic in a few aspects. A pandemic affects a wider geographical area, often worldwide and involves a larger number of people. It's often caused by a new virus or a new strain of virus that has not circulated within people for a long time. Being novel, humans have little to no immunity against the virus, and it spreads quickly causing more deaths.

Owing to its vast impact, it creates social disruption and economic loss.

The terms pandemic and epidemic are never used to indicate the severity of the disease, only the degree at which the disease is spreading.

COVID-19 Virus, an overview

Coronavirus is a family of viruses, which can cause the common cold or more severe diseases such as Severe Acute Respiratory Syndrome (SARS), or the Middle East Respiratory Syndrome (MERS), and the new corona virus disease COVID-19, that first appeared in late 2019 in Wuhan. This outbreak of corona virus initiated as pneumonia of unknown cause in December 2019 in Wuhan, China, which spread rapidly out of Wuhan to other countries.

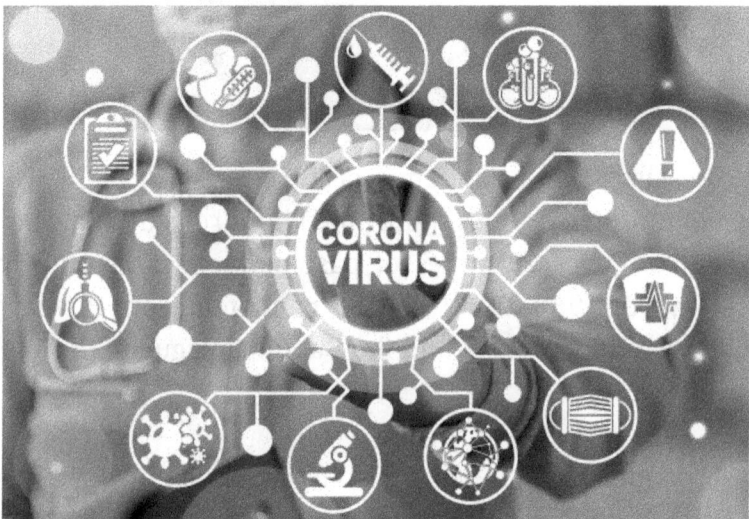

On 30th January 2020, the World Health Organization (WHO) declared the COVID-19 outbreak as the sixth public health emergency of international concern (PHEIC), and on 11th March 2020, the WHO announced COVID-19 as a pandemic. The COVID-19 pandemic has resulted in more than 73.9 million people becoming infected globally (at 17th December 2020) and has claimed the lives of more than 1.65 million people around the world (at 17th December 2020). The United States has the largest number of cases in the world — over 17.1 million (at 17th December 2020) — and more than 311,073 people have died (at 17th December 2020).

The exact incubation period is not known. It is presumed to be between 2 to 14 days after exposure, with most cases occurring within 5 days after exposure. The mode of spread of infection is through droplets. The virus is released in the respiratory secretions when an infected person coughs, sneezes or talks. These droplets can infect others if they make direct contact with the mucous membranes. Infection can also occur by touching an infected surface and followed by eyes, nose, or mouth. Droplets typically do not travel more than six feet (about two meters) and do not linger in the air. Patients are thought to be most contagious when they are symptomatic, but some spread might be possible before symptoms appear and in asymptomatic people.

The Infectious nature of COVID-19

This Novel corona virus is spread by people who have the virus coming in contact with people who are not infected. The more you come into contact with infected people, the more likely you are to catch the infection. Social distancing is infection control action that can be taken by public health officials to stop or slow down the spread of a highly contagious disease.

In addition to social distancing measures taken by governments, we can choose to reduce physical exposure to potentially sick people ourselves, for example, by exploring the option to work from home if your job allows for it. Avoiding large public gatherings such as sporting events or situations where you may come in to contact with crowds of people, for example, in busy shopping malls may help limit the spread of disease. People should be encouraged to interact with people over the phone/video calls, instead of in person.

Another step to minimize the risk of catching the disease is frequent hand washing for 20-40 seconds with soap and water. If soap and water are not available, the use of an alcohol-based hand sanitizer with at least 60% alcohol helps kill the germs and reduces chances of disease transmission. Given how often we use our phones, regularly sanitizing our phones seems like the next logical priority. Using antibacterial wipes or alcohol swabs (typically 70% alcohol) to clean your phone and other items is a measure to avoid the spread of the virus. We should all Sanitize other items we touch regularly including computer keyboard and mouse, house and car keys, re-usable water bottle etc. Sanitizing car steering wheel, door handles, switches, shelves, arms chairs, and other high touch surfaces is also necessary to avoid catching the virus.

The immune system plays a vital role in catching the infection and the severity of the illness. Keeping your immune system healthy helps you beat the virus. To do so, you should take adequate high-quality sleep at least for 7-8 hours, eat healthy, including high-quality proteins fruits vegetables and keep yourself hydrated. Active lifestyle, maintaining a healthy weight, and moderate exercise also contributes to your immune system and should be part of your daily routine to remain fit.

In a community, the spread of the virus can be minimized by adopting small steps like diligent hand washing, particularly after touching surfaces in public. If hands are not visibly dirty, a hand sanitizer that contains at least 60 per cent alcohol is a reasonable alternative. Respiratory hygiene (e.g., covering the cough or sneeze) limits the spread of diseases by containment of droplets that may carry virus particles if a person is infected. It is preferable to use a triple-layer disposable surgical mask if there are any respiratory symptoms or you are in a crowded place. Avoiding crowds (particularly in poorly ventilated spaces) if possible and avoiding close contact with ill individuals and maintaining a safe distance of at least 1 metre decreases your chances of getting infected. When meeting people avoid handshakes, hugs, and kisses. Avoiding non-essential travel and gatherings will result in fewer chances of infection. People should be advised to avoid holding onto the hand-railings of steps and either use pens or sanitize their hands after switching on lights in common areas and touching lift buttons to avoid getting their hands contaminated.

Commons symptoms of COVID-19 infection

The spectrum of COVID-19 severity varies from asymptomatic to mild self-limiting illness in most cases. In a few patients, it causes more severe illness or critical disease, particularly in the elderly population or in patients with underlying medical problems.

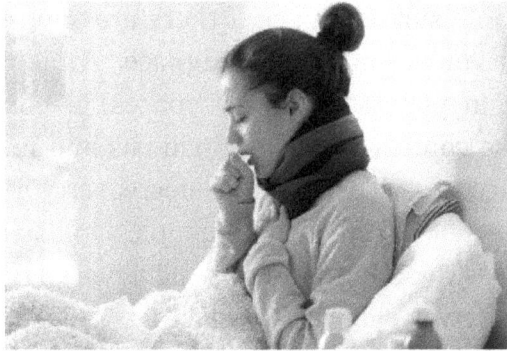

Most common symptoms are fever, cough, and shortness of breath. Some people complain of fatigue, body aches and pains, loss of sense of taste and smell and diarrhoea. Some develop rashes on their hands or feet. Pneumonia appears to be the most common and severe manifestation of infection. In severe illness, patients have hypoxemia (low levels of oxygen in the blood) and lung involvement visible on X-ray or CT imaging. A small percentage of people develop a critical disease ending up in acute respiratory distress, respiratory failure, shock and multi-organ dysfunction with a high mortality rate.

Clinical Classification of Disease

Asymptomatic
SARS CoV2 infection with no symptoms

Mild
- Presence of symptoms suggestive of COVID-19
- Stable vital signs (Blood pressure, arterial pulse, breathing rate, temperature)
- None OR minimal X-Ray findings
- Oxygen saturation equal or less than 93% at room air

Moderate
- Presence of symptoms suggestive of COVID-19
- Oxygen saturation less than 93% but great than 90% on room air
- Chest X-ray with infiltrates involving greater than 50% of the lung fields
- No complications and manifestations related to severe condition

Severe
In adults, clinical features suggestive of pneumonia and any of the following:

- Breathing rate less than 30/min
- Oxygen saturation equal to or less than 90% on room air
- Chest X-ray with infiltrates involving greater than 50% of lung fields

Critical

Any of the three manifestations

- Adult Respiratory Distress Syndrome – Moderate to Severe breathing trouble
- Multiorgan dysfunction – Involvement of many organs of the body
- Septic Shock – Significant drop of blood pressure due to spreading infection

ATYPICAL PRESENTATION IN COVID-19

Patients with COVID-19 may not have respiratory symptoms at presentation. Older people and immunosuppressed patients, in particular, may present with atypical symptoms such as fatigue, decreased alertness, reduced mobility, diarrhoea, loss of appetite, delirium, and absence of fever.

Others may have life-threatening conditions such as acute coronary syndrome, myocarditis, acute pulmonary embolism, and acute stroke. In many cases, neurological, eye and skin manifestation have been reported without respiratory symptoms.

Criteria for admission of COVID-19 patients

Asymptomatic (without symptoms) and Mild disease
Asymptomatic and mild cases can be managed at home or isolation facility.

Moderate, Severe and Critical disease

Patients with the above categories should be admitted to a hospital for further management.

- Moderate disease: Admit to a well-ventilated isolation ward with oxygen and monitoring facilities.
- Severe disease: Admit to high dependency unit (HDU)
- Critical disease: Admit to Intensive Care Unit (ICU)

At the moment, the therapeutic strategies to deal with the infection are only supportive, and prevention aimed at reducing transmission in the community is our best weapon:

Prophylaxis (Prevention of disease)

There is no proven role of prophylactic chloroquine or hydroxychloroquine or any other drug at this time.

There is no specific treatment for COVID-19 infection including Chloroquine, Hydroxychloroquine, Ivermectin, Famotidine, Montelukast, Colchicine (or any other drug or therapy in October 2020).

Mild disease

Mild cases should be treated with supportive care only, which includes the use of Acetaminophen for fever, oral hydration in case of diarrhoea and antihistamines for cough and sore throat.

Moderate, Severe, and Critical disease

Patients with moderate disease should receive supportive therapy. All patients must be assessed for the Cytokine Release Syndrome (CRS).

TREATMENT

I. OXYGEN

i. Oxygen therapy delivered in an escalating manner via nasal cannula, face mask and non-rebreather mask.

ii. Preference should be given to HFNC (High Flow Nasal Cannula) if available.

iii. Awake positioning the patient prone (face down) should be encouraged in cooperative patients.

II. ANTICOAGULATION

In admitted patients with severe or critical COVID-19 with high D-Dimer levels detected in the blood test.

III. STEROIDS

Administered in patients requiring oxygen or those with raised inflammatory markers like CRP.

IV. TOCILIZUMAB

Patients with evidence of Cytokine release syndrome may benefit from IL-6 blockers.

V. ANTIBIOTICS

Routine use of antibiotics is not recommended.

Antibiotics should only be used in cases where a bacterial infection is suspected. There is no role of prophylactic antibiotics to prevent secondary infection.

VI. CHLOROQUIN AND HYDROXICHLOROQUIN

There is a lack of clear-cut evidence at present for any benefit in COVID-19 patient.

VII.   ANTIVIRALS

Recent studies have shown encouraging results of Remdesivir in moderate and severe disease irrespective of the presence of CRS. It can also be given in critical cases; however, available data shows no benefit in critical cases.

VII.   CONVALESCENT PLASMA

Plasma therapy is still in the investigation stage and should be used cautiously as part of the clinical trial.

Investigational therapy

Treatment modalities including tocilizumab, convalescent plasma, antivirals, Ivermectin, Famotidine, Colchicine should be used only in the setting of a research protocol which includes consent and safety oversight.

Discontinuation of Isolation and Discharge from Hospital

Viral RNA shedding in COVID-19 declines with the resolution of symptoms and may continue for days to weeks. However, the detection of RNA during convalescence does not indicate the presence of a viable infectious virus. Isolation precautions can therefore be discontinued in the following conditions, and a test to document cure is not required in these patients.

SYMPTOMATIC PATIENTS WITH CONFIRMED COVID-19

In those who are SYMPTOMATIC, the following symptom-based strategy is recommended:

- At least ten days from the start of symptoms **AND**
- At least three days after resolution of symptoms (fever without antipyretics) and no or improved respiratory symptom, e.g., dry cough, shortness of breath).

ASYMPTOMATIC PATIENTS WITH CONFIRMED COVID-19

In those who are ASYMPTOMATIC, the following time-based strategy is recommended:

- Ten days from the date of the positive test

However, for the following categories of patients, two consecutive negative PCR tests 24 hours apart are required to discontinue isolation:

1. Immunocompromised patients
2. Healthcare workers involved in patient care
3. Those living in congregations such as hostels, madrasas, prisons, and community livings.

VACCINE FOR COVID 19

More than 180 vaccine candidates based on several different platforms are currently in development. The WHO maintains a working document that includes most of the vaccines in development and can be found online at the following web link:

https://www.who.int/publications/m/item/draft-landscape-of-COVID-19-candidate-vaccines.

The platforms can be divided into 'traditional' approaches like inactivated or live virus vaccines, platforms that have recently resulted in licensed vaccines (recombinant proteins, vectored vaccines) and platforms that have never been used for a licensed vaccine (RNA and DNA vaccines).

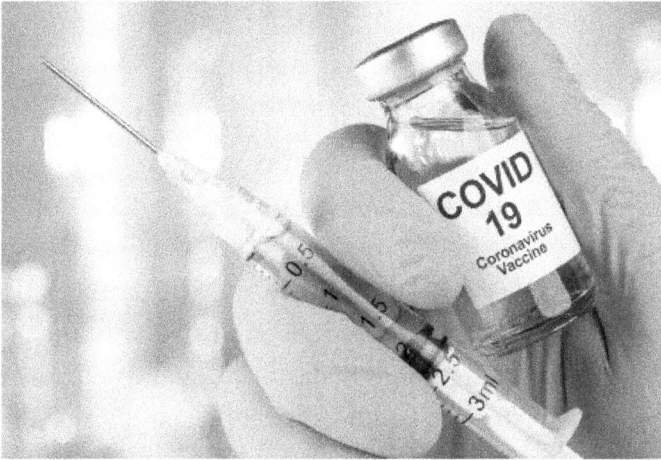

With nine vaccine candidates in Phase III trials already and encouraging data from many candidates in NHPs and Phase I, II or I/II trials, the situation can be described as cautiously positive. Some of the major questions including, duration of immunity of vaccine, efficacy in the elderly population, tolerability in children, rolling out and global distribution after licensing still remain unanswered. Despite all the challenges discussed above, the process of developing vaccines as a countermeasure against COVID-19 is at record speed, and it is certainly possible that vaccines with safety and efficacy proven in Phase III trials might already enter the market in 2020.

One vaccine from a Chinese company is already being used for phase three trials recruiting Pakistani population.

TELEMEDICINE and COVID-19

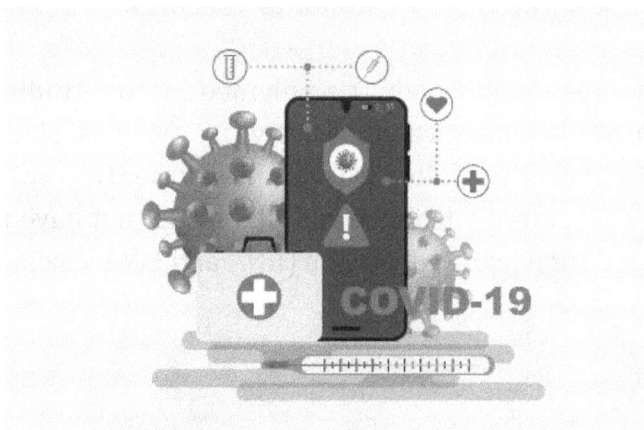

Natural disasters and epidemics pose many challenges in providing health care. COVID-19 was no different, and it caused unprecedented stress on health systems disrupting the health delivery system in the affected countries. Unique and innovative solutions were needed to maintain patient continuity and management of patients during COVID-19 and Telemedicine proved to be one such tool. It allows continuity of patient care while limiting exposure to virus among patients, healthcare workers and other hospital or clinic staff, which is critical in controlling the spread and transmission. The use of Telemedicine at the time of COVID-19 pandemic not only enabled management of disease but also helped in epidemiological research and control of the disease.

The use of Telemedicine technology was one of the initiatives taken by the health system in Pakistan in a public-private partnership. This twenty-first-century approach that is both patient-centred and protects patients and physicians, as well as others has proved to be of great benefit in successfully treating the patient by providing them with remote consultations making the use of technology. Telemedicine centres operating across the country worked 24/7 in making the public aware of disease symptoms, guiding them towards a testing facility, explaining warning signs and facilitating referral to hospitals when needed. With this new health care delivery system people were categorized not only according to disease severity based on a simple scoring system but also on many occasions treated by consultants by video consultation and monitoring.

During the pandemic, many medical universities set up Telemedicine centers to benefit patients. The project was initiated at the University of Health Sciences, Lahore Pakistan through the Doctors 24/7 Online Telemedicine website, followed by replication of the service by several Medical Institutions in the province of Punjab. King Edward Medical University also contributed significantly by setting up a Skype-based Video Consultation system to support the healthcare initiative.

The University of Health Sciences adopted the Telemedicine Helpline service through the www.Doctors247. online Telemedicine software (Medical City Online's proprietary software) by developing the Central Hub at University premises with an alternative backup Telephone line as well. The Telemedicine Helpline operating 24/7 to provide free medical advice was well adopted and received at outpatient clinics in both public hospitals and private sector, lessening the unnecessary burden in the hospitals and clinics. It enabled the delivery of healthcare services by health care professionals, where distance was a critical factor, through using information and communication technologies for the exchange of valid and correct information. With the rapid evolution and downsizing of portable electronics, most families have at least one digital device, such as a smartphone or webcam that could provide communication between patient and healthcare provider.

Video conferencing and similar television systems were also used to provide healthcare programs for people who were hospitalized or in quarantine to reduce the risk of exposure to others and employees. Physicians who were looking after patients in quarantine employed these services to take care of their patients remotely. In addition, covering multiple sites with a Tele-physician could address some of the challenges of the workforce who were also severely affected by COVID-19.

There are various additional benefits in using the technology of Telemedicine. Apart from COVID-19, regular outpatient consultations for the patients were also affected. New Telemedicine care for non-emergency and routine cases were offered Telemedicine consultations while services that did not require direct patient-provider interaction, such as providing psychological services or follow-up care of chronic medical conditions like Diabetes, Hypertension, Tuberculosis etc., were also shifted to Teleconsultations.

Remote care reduced the use of resources within health centres, improved access to care while minimizing the risk of direct transmission of the infectious agent from person to person. In addition to being beneficial in keeping people safe, another important advantage was providing wide access to medical services and to caregivers. Therefore, this technology proved to be an attractive, effectual, and affordable option in the current pandemic.

With every new technology come some limitations. Lack of infrastructure and technology specific to Telemedicine in remote settings, regulatory and other issues proved to be a major barrier in some health facilities, but with political will and support from government policies, these were overcome.

About the Chapter Author

Dr Somia Iqtadar FCPS

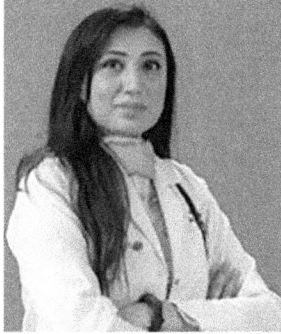

D r Somia Iqtadar is an immensely capable and accomplished young doctor working in the capacity of an Associate Professor of Medicine at King Edward Medical University (KEMU).

Her contributory role to healthcare of Pakistan is well reflected by her various appointments such as Chairperson Dengue Expert Advisory Group Punjab, Member of Technical working Group on Corona and also Corona Expert Advisory Group Punjab.

She is also the first General Secretary of Pakistan Society of Internal Medicine. She has numerous publications in indexed national as well as international journals of high impact factor. She is the primary author of Government of Central Punjab (GCP) guidelines on Dengue, H1N1 and COVID-19 in Pakistan.

Recently, Dr Somia Iqtadar has been awarded Laurels of Honour Award by Women Chamber of Commerce & Industry and Governor Punjab as "COVID Hero Woman of the Year in Health 2020". Due to her immense interest in medical education and accomplishments, she was selected as a member of the international advisory board as an author in the famed and well recognised medical textbook Kumar and Clark Textbook of Medicine, wherein she contributed in its latest edition by authoring three important chapters on Dengue, Congo and Ebola. She has also written a book for the general public on Dengue and is a contributing author in an international book on the role of Telehealth in COVID management in Pakistan.

Being an adept orator and presenter, she has represented Pakistan in numerous international conferences, presenting her research and experiences. Her areas of interest include cardiometabolic medicine, infectious diseases, and Telehealth. She has also been nominated in top 100 women in global health in Pakistan chapter.

Dr Somia Iqtadar primarily authored the first Edition of COVID-19 Guideline and SOPs of Govt of Punjab Feb 2020. She was nominated as a member of Corona Expert Advisory Group in March 2020. Due to her tireless and diligent services, she was able to conduct Training of CEOs Health on COVID-19 Prevention and Control May 2020.

Furthermore, she actively engaged in and formulated Quarantine and Home isolation guidelines which were presented to Chief secretary health Punjab including all DCs in May 2020. She also conducted and facilitated First Press Briefing of CEAG and TWG 22nd June 2020 and has accompanied Honourable Minister of health in many Press briefings.

Dr Somia Iqtadar is an active member of, and leading as well as contributing in, different research projects related to COVID-19 across Pakistan; being an active member of King Edward Medical University Pakistan Research Board on COVID-19. Because of her ardent aptitude, she was able to enrol the maximum number of patients (115) in PROTECT trial, a multi-centre state of the art trial for the treatment of COVID-19 and is actively involved in national and collaborative international research projects related to COVID-19.

Chapter Eight

International Comparisons of the Corona virus Pandemic and the Rate of COVID-19 infection

Authors: Prof W Angus Wallace and Dr Rana Jawad Asghar

Coronavirus disease, now named COVID-19 by the World Health Organisation is a highly infectious disease caused by a new corona-virus (SARS-CoV-2) that is believed to have spontaneously surfaced in Wuhan, China in November 2019. In this chapter, we will explore how badly three countries – Pakistan, the United Kingdom (UK) and the United States of America (USA) were affected by COVID-19. Each of these countries dealt with the pandemic differently and started their lockdowns at different times. At the time of completing this book (February 2021), all three countries had experienced a first wave of the pandemic and were still recovering from their second wave.

It has been tough to carry out an analysis comparing the three countries because of the different definitions used for COVID-19 deaths, the difference in testing rates between the three countries and the inevitable inaccuracies that occurred in the first months of the epidemic within each of the countries as they tried to come to grips with the signs and symptoms of the disease, a lack of early testing facilities and missed diagnoses.

The severity of the Coronavirus pandemic has been quantified in a number of ways, but the most straightforward metrics we are using for comparison are 1) The daily number of new cases/million population of COVID-19; 2) The daily number of new COVID-19 associated deaths/

million population and 3) The national excess deaths/ million population that has occurred in each of these countries during the period of the COVID-19 pandemic. Unfortunately, comparisons are not easy because different types of tests with different accuracy were available in these three countries. Access to testing was widely different with varying criteria for testing, particularly at the early stages of the pandemic.

There is also an issue of different methodologies and definitions of what will constitute a death from COVID-19. Pakistan especially does not have a good vital statistics system, so deaths outside hospitals are not recorded unless there is a legal requirement. Not all hospital deaths are recorded as COVID 19 deaths due to classification differences. However, it is still very valuable to look at these comparisons but with these caveats in the forefront of our mind.

8.1 Definitions and Tests Used to Monitor COVID-19 in Pakistan, the UK, Europe & the USA

1) Daily number of new reported cases

This would seem to be the most straightforward metric to collect, but it has turned out to be remarkably difficult.

This is for many reasons – initially, there was no reliable test for an acute infection; then the tests became more readily available, but their accuracy was questioned; then the method of taking the swabs for active infections was highlighted as being important with poor swabbing techniques meaning many cases were missed, and more recently saliva tests that generally have an 80% to 90% accuracy.

The daily number of new cases has also been challenging to ascertain because up to 50% of new cases are symptom-free, but the infected person carries the virus and can infect others while they are actively infected.

Access to testing is another area which needs to be factored in before making comparison among countries. If a country is doing more testing, they will invariably identify more cases, especially when around 50% are asymptomatic. However, if a country is testing fewer numbers and only symptomatic cases, they will be missing much more cases.

Figure 8.1 – Daily new confirmed cases of COVID-10 and COVID-19 Associated Deaths in Pakistan, the UK & the USA from February to 16th November 2020 (Extracted from the WHO Coronavirus Disease (COVID-19) Dashboard - Please note difference in scales)

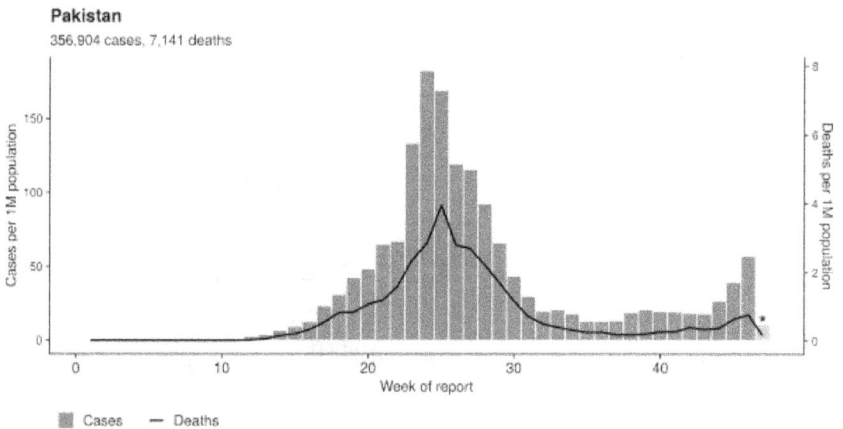

United Kingdom of Great Britain and Northern Ireland

1,369,322 cases, 51,934 deaths

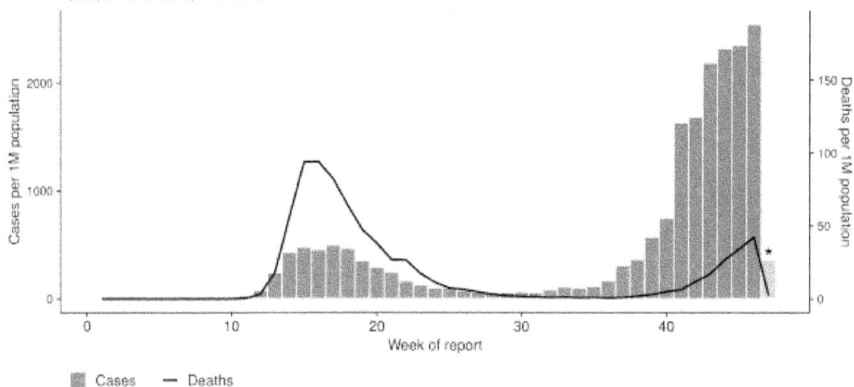

United States of America

10,796,432 cases, 243,758 deaths

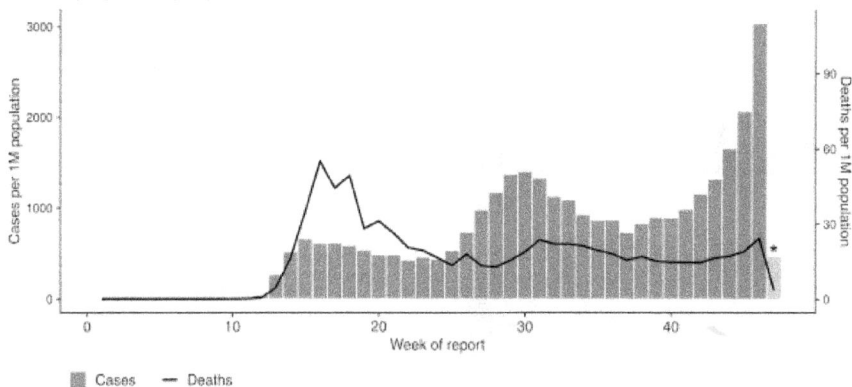

Figure 8.2 – Comparison of New confirmed cases of COVID-19 in Pakistan, the UK & the USA from February to 16th November 2020 (Extracted from the WHO Coronavirus Disease (COVID-19) Dashboard)

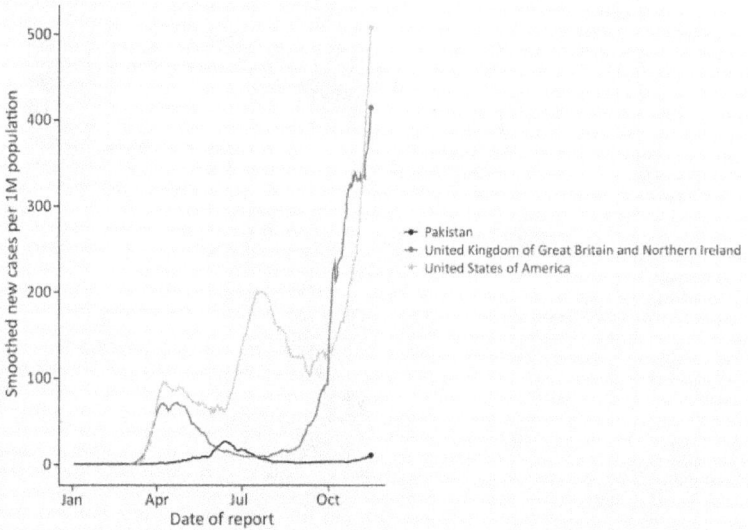

Data taken from COVID Intel database on 2020-11-17.
The line and associated text show the trend in incidence of COVID-19 cases.

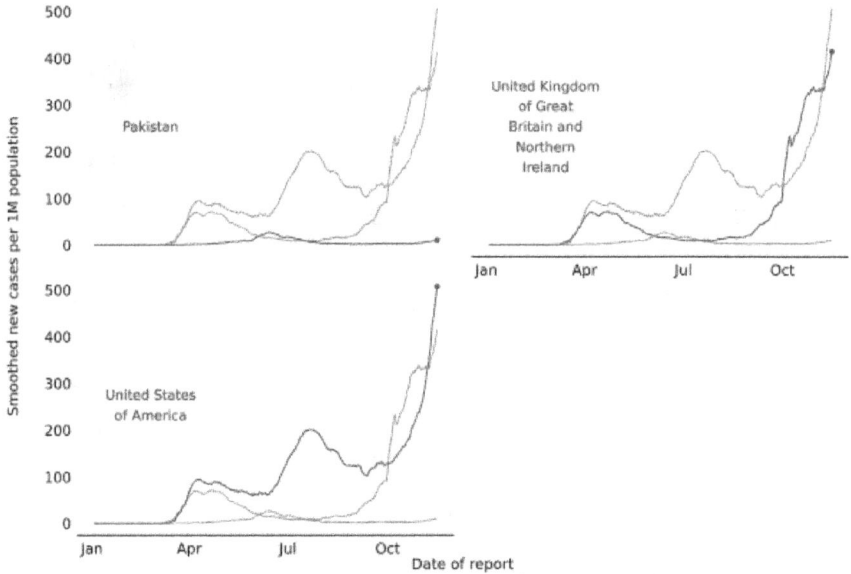

Data taken from COVID Intel database on 2020-11-17.
The lines and associated text show the trend in incidence of COVID-19 cases.

Figure 8.3 – Comparison of Deaths from COVID-10 in Pakistan, the UK & the USA from February to 16th November 2020 (Extracted from the WHO Coronavirus Disease (COVID-19) Dashboard)

Excess mortality during COVID-19: The number of deaths from all causes compared to previous years, all ages

Shown is how the number of weekly deaths in 2020 differs (as a percentage) from the average number of deaths in the same week over the previous five years (2015-2020). This metric is called the P-score. We do not show data from the most recent weeks because it is incomplete due to delays in death reporting.

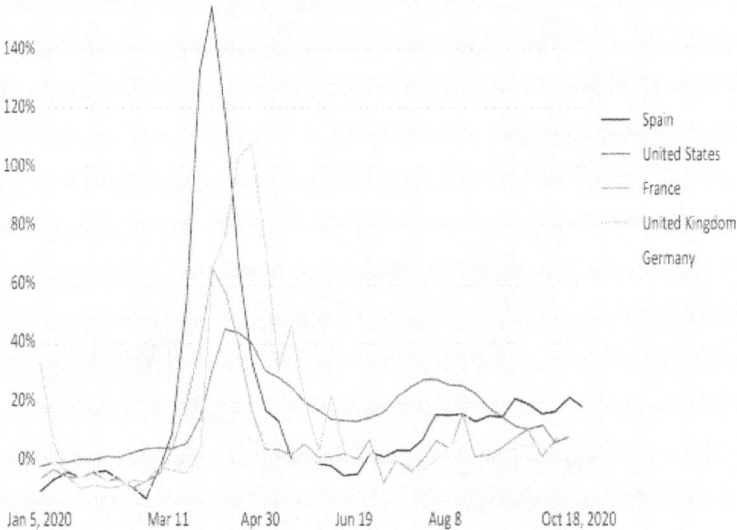

Source: Human Mortality Database (2020), UK Office for National Statistics (2020)
Note: Dates refer to the last day in each reporting week for most but not all countries. More details can be found in the Sources tab.
OurWorldInData.org/coronavirus • CC BY

8.2) Daily number of reported COVID-19 Associated Deaths

COVID-19 Associated Deaths are listed above in Figures 8.1, 8.2 & 8.3. They have been defined differently by different countries, and some have actually changed with time. **Table 8.1** shows the definitions used when they were changed, and the different ways the numbers have been counted – this has been a significant cause for confusion. However, any comparison among different countries must always be standardised by their population; otherwise, a country with a bigger population will have more cases even if both countries have the same case rate.

Table 8.1 – Definitions for COVID-19 Associated Deaths for Pakistan, the UK & the USA.

Country	Dates covered	Definition
Pakistan	March 2020 >	Death in a person with a laboratory-confirmed positive COVID-19 test and died within (equal to or less than) 21 days of the first positive specimen date (cause of death might not be due to COVID-19).
UK* (daily deaths)	Before 12th August 2020 (England only)	Death in a person with a laboratory-confirmed positive COVID-19 test who has subsequently died (cause of death might not be due to COVID-19).
UK* (daily deaths)	From 12th August 2020 (England only) December 2019 > (Rest of the UK – Scotland + Wales + Northern Ireland)	Death in a person with a laboratory-confirmed positive COVID-19 test and died within (equal to or less than) 28 days of the first positive specimen date will now be reported (cause of death might not be due to COVID-19).
UK* (weekly deaths)	Office for National Statistics (ONS) * Reference – www.kingsfund.org.uk/ publications/deaths-COVID-19	The ONS provides figures weekly based on deaths certified and registered in England and Wales with COVID-19 as an underlying or contributory cause of death (i.e., all 'mentions' of COVID-19 on death certificates). The figures include all COVID-19 deaths, in all settings, whether tested for COVID-19 or suspected by the certifying doctor based on the deceased's symptoms. ONS data has a reporting delay of 11 days from the date of death due to processes around death certification and registration.
EU	December 2019 > www.ecdc.europa.eu/en/COVID-19/surveillance/surveillance-definitions	A COVID-19 death is defined for surveillance purposes as a death resulting from a clinically compatible illness in a probable or confirmed COVID-19 case unless there is a clear alternative cause of death that cannot be related to COVID disease (e.g. trauma)
USA	December 2019 > Reference – www.cdc.gov/nchs/data/ nvss/vsrg/vsrg03-508.pdf	If COVID–19 played a role in the death, this condition should be specified on the death certificate. In many cases, it is likely that it will be the underlying cause of death (UCOD), as it can lead to various life-threatening conditions, such as pneumonia and acute respiratory distress syndrome (ARDS). In these cases, COVID–19 should be reported on the lowest line used in Part I with the other conditions to which it gave rise listed on the lines above it.

Because death can normally only be a confirmed death if confirmed by a COVID-19 test, the number of available tests in each country is important.

The less the number of tests per thousand people, the more likely COVID-19 deaths will have occurred but are not picked up. Because of the limited number of tests available in Pakistan, they will have an inaccurate and far lower incidence of confirmed COVID-19 deaths.

Figure 8.4 – Daily COVID-19 Testing rates in Pakistan, the UK & the USA from February to 16th November 2020 - Extracted from WHO Corona virus Disease (COVID-19) Dashboard

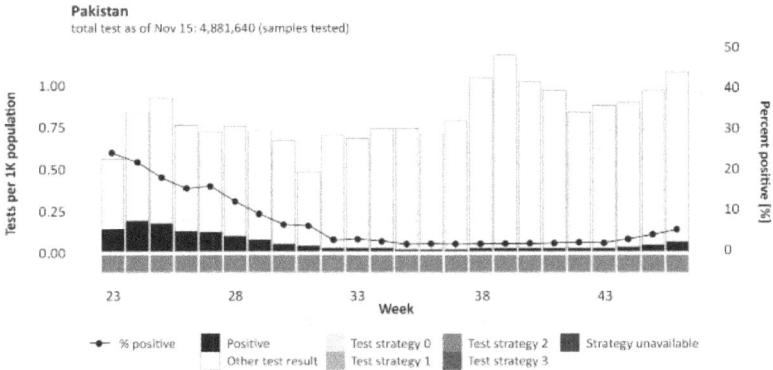

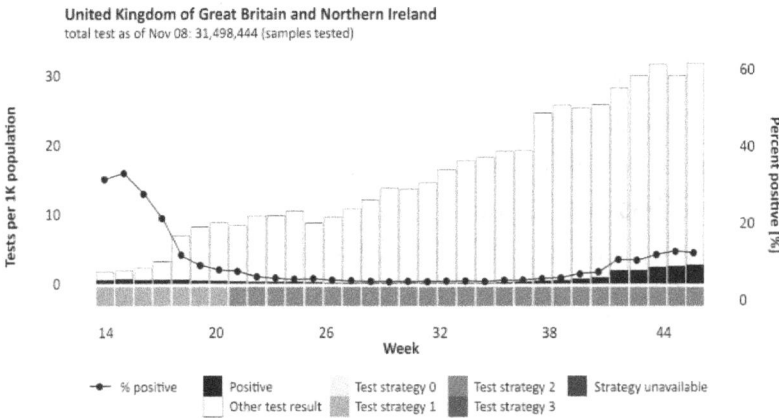

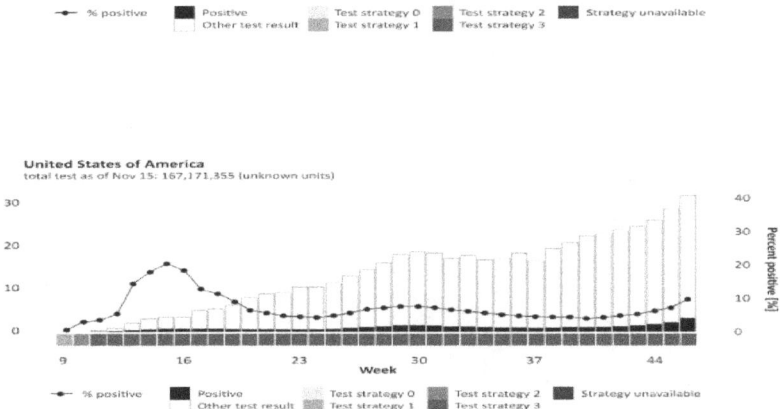

Testing index: The testing index is made up of two dimensions:
1. Testing rate - 4 point scale:
   1 = 0.0 - 0.5 tests per 1000 in past week
   2 = 0.51 - 1.0 tests per 1000 in past week
   3 = 1.01 - 3.0 tests per 1000 in past week
   4 = >3.01 tests per 1000 in past week
2. Testing strategy - 4 point scale
   0 = No testing strategy
   1 = Only those who both (a) have symptoms AND (b) meet specific criteria
   2 = Anyone showing symptoms

8.3 Weekly number of Total Excess Deaths

Because of the international lack of uniformity relating to the methods of detecting and identifying new cases and the differences in the definition of COVID-19 associated deaths, many epidemiologists now believe that the most reliable figures available for assessing the mortality associated with COVID-19 is the metric of "Weekly Excess Deaths in the population".

This has been applied successfully for 2020 for the United Kingdom and many other European countries.

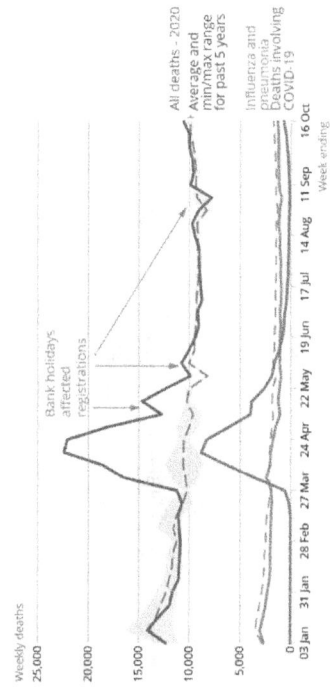

Figure 1: Deaths in England and Wales involving COVID-19 increased for the sixth consecutive week

Number of deaths registered by week, England and Wales, 28 December 2019 to 16 October 2020

Source: Office for National Statistics

Notes:

1. Figures include deaths of non-residents.

2. Based on date a death was registered rather than occurred.

3. All figures for 2020 are provisional.

4. The International Classification of Diseases, Tenth Edition (ICD-10) definitions are as follows: coronavirus (COVID-19) (U07.1 and U07.2) and Influenza and Pneumonia (J09-J18).

5. A death can be registered with both COVID-19 and Influenza and Pneumonia mentioned on the death certificate. Because pneumonia may be a consequence of COVID-19, deaths where both were mentioned have been counted only in the COVID-19 category.

6. Figures for Influenza and Pneumonia represent where either of these causes have been mentioned anywhere on the death certificate meaning they will not necessarily be the underlying cause of death.

7. The number of deaths registered in Weeks 19, 20, 22, 23, 36 and 37 were impacted by the Early May, Late May and August Bank Holidays (Friday 8 May 2020 in Week 19, Monday 25 May 2020 in Week 22 and Monday 31 August 2020); the impact of the Early May Bank Holiday was analysed in our Week 20 bulletin.

Figure 8.3b Total Excess deaths from any cause in various European Countries from February to June 2020 extracted from https://www.health.org.uk/news-and-comment/ charts-and-infographics/comparing-COVID-19-impact-in-the-uk-to-european-countries

Weekly excess deaths for selected European countries
Change from baseline weekly deaths, by week, 2020

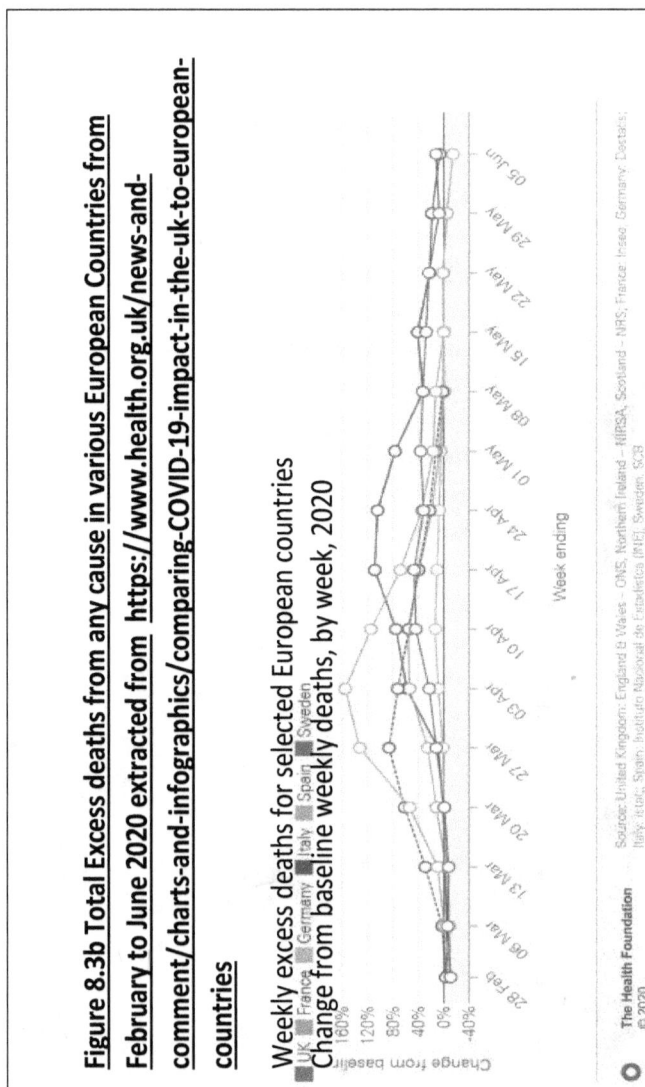

Figure 8.3c Total Excess deaths from any cause in the USA
www.cdc.gov/mmwr/volumes/69/wr/mm6942e2.htm

FIGURE 1. Weekly numbers of deaths from all causes and from all causes excluding COVID-19 relative to the
average expected number and the upper bound of the 95% prediction interval (A), and the weekly and total
numbers of deaths from all causes and from all causes excluding COVID-19 above the average expected number
and the upper bound of the 95% prediction interval (B) — National Vital Statistics System, United States,
January–September 2020

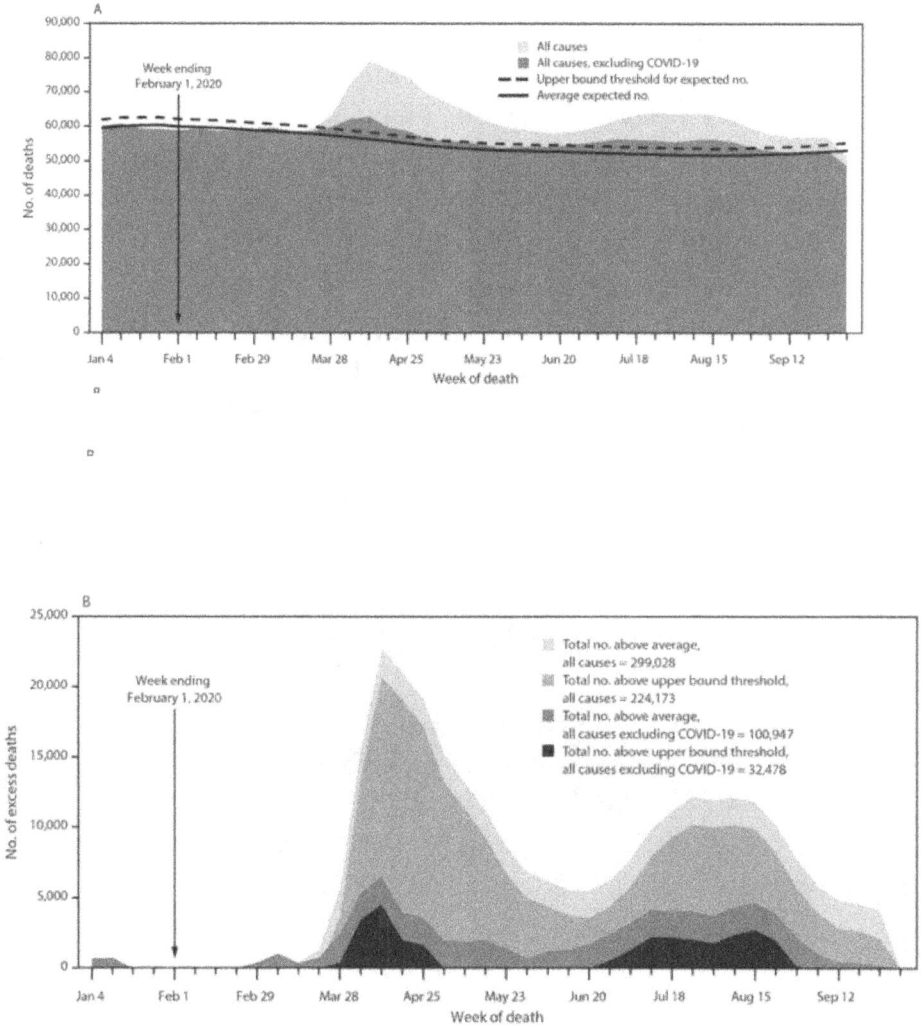

Abbreviation: COVID-19 = coronavirus disease 2019.

Data obtained by the BBC from officials in Pakistan's two largest cities, Karachi and Lahore, show that there was a significant rise in graveyard burials in June 2020 that can't be explained by corona virus deaths alone. For example, in Miani Sahib graveyard, the largest in Lahore, in June 2020 there were 1,176 burials this June, compared to 696 in June last year.

Only 48 of the burials this June were of officially recorded coronavirus patients. The rise is likely to be a combination of undetected corona virus deaths, and patients suffering from other illnesses not getting treatment as hospitals were under such pressure.

www.bbc.com/news/world-asia-53742214

Because it has been so difficult to establish the number of excess deaths in 2020/21 in Pakistan, the authors are currently exploring the registers for burials in Pakistan that will provide more accurate figures for excess deaths with a view to these being published in a later edition of this book.

Summary statistical comparisons

The other factors that need to be considered when carrying out national comparisons are the population size, the land area covered by the country, the population density and the proportion of urban and rural areas in the different countries. These are compared in Table 8.2 below.

Table 8.2 – Population size, Land Area, Urbanisation and COVID-19 Associated Confirmed Infections and Deaths in Pakistan, the UK and the USA

Data taken from WHO COVID Intel database in February 2021

Country	Population size	Land Area (Km^2)	Population density (/km^2)	Urban (Km^2)	Total COVID-19 New cases	COVID-19 New cases /million population	Total COVID-19 Associated Deaths	COVID-19 Associated Deaths/million population
Pakistan	220,892,340	881,913	250	35,872	549,032	2,486	11,802	53.4
UK	67,886,011	242,495	280	17,700	3,852,627	56,751	108,013	1,591.0
USA	331,002,651	9,158,064	36	63,400	26,172,274	79,070	443,256	1,339.1

Figures 8.1, 8.2 and 8.3 show the histograms extracted from the WHO Corona virus Disease (COVID-19) Dashboard, which records all the data relating to Corona virus incidence and fatalities supplied individually from each country.

Reviewing the data in Figures 8.1 to 8.3, Pakistan appears to have been more successful than both the UK and the USA in controlling their Coronavirus epidemic. However, Pakistan COVID-19 testing has been very low compared to the other two comparison countries. At 4th February 2021, the number of Coronavirus tests reported (both for acute infection and past infection) by Pakistan = 8,041,254, by the UK = 71,642,534 and by the USA = 310,683,694. Because of the discrepancies in Coronavirus testing it is important to calculate the number of tests per 1 million population - for Pakistan = 36,403, for the UK = 1,055,336 and for the USA = 938,614. Because Pakistan has carried out far fewer tests per million population they will inevitably underestimate their Coronavirus associated deaths.

8.4. The Risk of infection and Death to Health Care Staff in Pakistan, the UK and the USA

The risk of infection and death to Health Care Staff in Pakistan, the UK and the USA has been revealed in an Amnesty International report which has identified Health Care Staff fatalities in Pakistan at 58 (by early July 2020) www.thenews.com.pk/print/680655-pakistan-has-lost-42-doctors-among-58-healthcare-providers-to-COVID-19; in the UK at 540 and in the USA at 507.

By 3rd September 2020 the UK mortality for Healthcare workers had risen to 649 and the US mortality for Healthcare workers was 1,077.

However, later reports from the Pakistan National Emergency Operations Centre (NEOC), revealed that 6,995 Healthcare Workers (HCWs) had been infected with the COVID-19 so far and 78 had died. https://nation.com.pk/29-Aug-2020/over-6-000-healthcare-workers-infected-with-coronavirus-in-country. This is clearly, far less than those affected in the UK and USA.

The covid-19 pandemic continues to take a harsh toll on healthcare workers. In the Mirror newspaper on 20 January 2021: "52,000 NHS staff are off sick with covid." (Glaze, B 2021). Over 850 UK healthcare workers are thought to have died of covid between March and December 2020; at least 3000 have died in the US. (Shone E, 2021) (The Guardian, 2021)

Our Hypotheses

It is very difficult to ascertain with accuracy all the reasons why Pakistan appears to have fared better in this COVID-19 pandemic (up to February 2021).

Hypothesis 1 (RJA)

One important factor relating to the low Pakistan death figures is the population age profile in Pakistan. RJA is a leading Pakistani epidemiologist. He believes the principal reason for the low mortality rate is Pakistan's young population. The average age of the population in Pakistan is 22 years, compared to about 41 in the UK. The vast majority of deaths globally from the Coronavirus have been of elderly patients.

Dr Asghar told the BBC on 20th August 2020 that less than 4% of Pakistan's population is aged 65 and above, whereas in more developed countries the proportion is around 20-25%. "That is why we haven't seen that many deaths in Pakistan," he said.

www.bbc.co.uk/news/world-asia-53742214.

Another factor, Dr Asghar said, was that social circles in developing world countries are smaller than the West. "Once a virus has run out of those social circles which are intermixing, it dies down," he said. Dr Asghar told the BBC that tracking systems needed to be improved in order to detect new spikes in cases. The fact that Pakistan had so far done better than feared "does not mean we are out of danger", he said.

We consider Hypothesis 1 to by highly likely but not proven.

Hypothesis 2 (WAW & SC)

The early introduction, in mid-March 2020, of the Corona Telemedicine Service supported by both the State of Punjab and nationally by the Prime Minister, meant that patients who experienced any concerns or symptoms did not attend their family doctor or the hospital but instead made direct contact with the online Corona Service by either using their mobile phone, tablet or laptop or asking a family member to do so for them.

Over 500,000 Telemedicine consultations were held. If we assume that half of these (250,000 patients) could have been patients with Coronavirus infections, then the Telemedicine service has resulted in reducing the clinical contact between these patients and health service staff by 250,000 with the consequent avoidance of cross-infection and the need for PPE equipment for these contacts.

We consider Hypothesis 2 to by highly likely but not proven.

Hypothesis 3 (WAW & SC)

Coronavirus transmission cannot take place through a Telemedicine consultation using either phones or computers. The virus cannot travel along phone lines, nor can it be transmitted using Bluetooth or Wi-fi.

We consider that Hypothesis 3 is correct and proven.

Hypothesis 4 (WAW & SC)

The use of Telemedicine and, in particular, the Doctors24/7 Corona Telemedicine Service has resulted in a reduction of COVID-19 infections, transmission of disease and the cross-infection of health care staff in Pakistan.

One factor we have considered is that for both patients and healthcare staff in Pakistan, early use of modern technology and, in particular, the nationwide use of the Corona Telemedicine service that was launched early in the epidemic (on 15th March 2020).

The Corona Telemedicine platform provided smart-phone video communication between the general public and the nationally appointed and trained Telemedicine Advisors. This provided reassurance for the general public, but also provided the facility for a "face-to-face" Corona Score to be completed that then facilitated triage of patients. This undoubtedly reduced the number of patients attending the doctors and hospitals and removed the risk of healthcare staff infection with Coronavirus.

Although we consider this is highly likely, we have been unable to identify definite evidence to support this hypothesis, so it remains not proven.

8.5 The Corona Telemedicine timeline summarised (for reference)

1) On 15th March 2020, the Medical City Online Telemedicine platform was released by the Pakistan Government for field testing in Pakistan and doctors were invited to volunteer to help with Telemedicine management of Pakistan patients (see attached).

2) On 18th March 2020, the Pakistan government announced that field testing had been successful, and the Telemedicine platform was to be rolled out across the whole of Pakistan (attached).

3) The Pakistan Telemedicine platform and the Corona Advisers can be seen at https://doctors247.online.

4) On 15th August 2020, Dr Suhail Chughtai's Telemedicine software design related work was given national recognition in the form of Foreign Office awards through a virtual ceremony at the Pak High Commission London office.

5) On 28th August 2020, Professor Suhail Chughtai received a national Pakistan honour by Ch. Muhammad Sarwar, Governor of Punjab for his contribution to the development of the National UHS Telemedicine Centre.

References

(WHO), W.H.O. *Coronavirus disease (COVID-19) pandemic. 2020; Available from https://www.who.int/emergencies/diseases/novel-coronavirus-2019.*

Amnesty_International, *Exposed, Silenced, Attacked: Failures to protect health and essential workers during the pandemic. 2020. p. 61.*

Ghosh, I., *Mapped: The Anatomy of Land Use in America, in Visual Capitalist. 2020.*

Mundi, I. *Urban land area (sq. km) - Pakistan. 2020; Available from https://www.indexmundi.com/facts/pakistan/indicator/AG.LND.TOTL.UR.K2.*

Statistics, O.O.f.N. *UK natural capital: urban accounts. 2020; Available from https://www.ons.gov.uk/economy/environmentalaccounts/bulletins/uknaturalcapital/urbanaccounts.*

Wikipedia. *United Kingdom. 2020; Available from https://en.wikipedia.org/wiki/United_Kingdom.*

Wikipedia. *Pakistan. 2020; Available from https://en.wikipedia.org/wiki/Pakistan.*

Wikipedia. *List of U.S. states and territories by area. 2020; Available from https://en.wikipedia.org/wiki/List_of_U.S._states_and_territories_by_area.*

WHO Coronavirus Disease (COVID-19) Dashboard

Amnesty International (2020) *Exposed, Silenced, Attacked: Failures To Protect Health And Essential Workers During The COVID-19 Pandemic. Index: POL 40/2572/2020 July 2020 amnesty.org*

Dr Rana Jawad Asghar

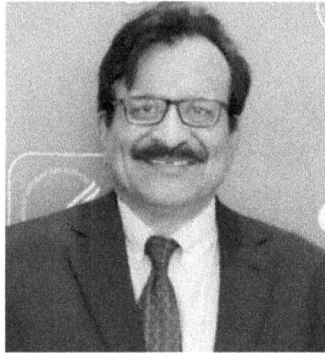

Dr Rana Jawad Asghar is Chief Executive officer of GHSI

(Global Health Strategists and Implementers) a consulting company in Pakistan. He is an adjunct professor of epidemiology at the University of Nebraska, USA and member of WHO Rooster of Experts in Epidemiology and Surveillance.

He was the fourth Pakistani to be selected in 60+ year history of Epidemic Intelligence Service, US CDC. He has served as a Program Manager for Child Survival Program in Mozambique, a faculty member at the London School of Hygiene and Tropical Medicine and Research Associate at the Stanford University, USA.

He set up Pakistan Field Epidemiology and Laboratory Training Program (FELTP) and Disease surveillance and response units (DSRU) as a US-CDC Resident Adviser working with the Government of Pakistan. https://www. linkedin.com/in/epidemiology/

Chapter Nine

Analysis of the Impact of the Telemedicine Helpline

Analysis of its wider National Impact beyond remote healthcare delivery

Author: Dr Suhail Chughtai

The Telemedicine Helpline, a phenomenon

This e-project engaged a large number of people including the Political Leaders such as the Governor of Punjab, Academicians such as the Vice Chancellors of most of the Punjab Medical Universities, Senior and Junior Doctors, Management staff at the Telemedicine Hubs, Media Personalities for campaigning, healthcare policymakers and more. Various objectives were met as summed up below:

- **Less crowding at Government Hospitals and Private Clinics**

    People rushing to medical facilities to seek advice for suspected Coronavirus infection could have flooded the Government hospitals and private clinics which was prevented by providing an alternative medical triage service through this Telemedicine website.

    The influx of patients and their attendants could have increased the COVID-19 infection burden by either transmitting or catching the virus through cross-infection, thus multiplying the epidemic many-fold. The Doctors 24/7 Online website was successful in keeping patients at home and out of crowded waiting rooms.

- **Reduced the Mortality and Morbidity of the people**

Telehealth is known to substantially reduce mortality, reduce the need for hospital admissions, lower the number of bed days spent in hospitals and reduce the time spent in emergency departments of both Government and private medical facilities.

Trials have shown that, if used correctly, Telehealth can deliver a 15% reduction in emergency room visits; a 20% reduction in emergency admissions; a 14% reduction in elective admissions; a 14% reduction in bed days; and an 8% reduction in tariff costs. More strikingly, the findings showed a 45% reduction in mortality rates. The overall effect of the Telemedicine project helped spare the hospital resources for the very needy ones thus the Outpatient spaces were not crowded during the critical phase of COVID-19 epidemic in Pakistan with ICU beds almost always available for the patients with breathing distress.

- **Increased safety of Healthcare Professionals**

Despite over 6000 healthcare workers getting infected with COVID-19, the number of deaths within the healthcare fraternity in Pakistan remained relatively low as compared to other countries including the UK. Pakistan lost 75 healthcare workers in the line of the duty to October 2020.

- **Opportunities to Evaluate of the Disease penetration in the community**

The Corona Score Form embedded in Doctors 24/7 Online helped understand the hot spots in the country, thus enabling a study of the disease burden and demographic distribution.

- **Reduced anxiety of the general public during periods of home-confinement**

  A number of emerging stories of patients calling not only from various cities in Pakistan but also from other countries such as UAE, Saudi Arabia, Qatar, Kuwait, reflected that patients felt relieved after having spoken to the doctor over a live teleconsultation. The mere stress of not being able to have access to a doctor was alleviated by having round-the-clock, free of charge, online medical advice.

- **Healthcare for Medical Conditions other than COVID-19 addressed**

  Common symptoms like abdominal pain, skin rashes, headaches, mild diarrhoea were also dealt with by the Telemedicine Helpline Healthcare providers, which again served the objectives well.

- **Educating the Patients and Public at large about Telemedicine**

  Telemedicine, despite being a relatively new modality, was accepted well under the pressure imposed by COVID-19 related social confinement which necessitated and accelerated the understanding of Telehealth.

- **Empowering the Medical Fraternity about Telemedicine**

  The medical fraternity, during the first phase of the COVID-19 pandemic gained confidence in the Telemedicine assisted delivery of care and they began to believe that "Telemedicine is going to be the medicine". The future evolution of healthcare services in Pakistan to equalise the physician density through Telemedicine got on the road to a fast-track evolution since doctors now feel more acquainted with the application and usefulness of Telemedicine.

- **Significant cost saving for the Punjab Health Department**

Setting up Telemedicine Hubs and connecting to patients via the website is less costly than setting up an Outpatient unit. Patients who visited Doctors 24/7 Online could meet a doctor for a Teleconsultation free of charge as well as having no travelling expenses. The Telemedicine Software was provided free of charge to the Government of Punjab by Medical City Online while the key front line healthcare professionals and the project management task force volunteered as a result of their commitment to the national call of duty.

- **To lower the disease burden on patients**

The Telemedicine helpline delivered around the clock providing free of charge medical advice in order to ease several burdens on a patient, especially during the stressful times of COVID-19 related circumstances:
  - The Logistic burden (Travelling to/from clinic)
  - The Social burden (Engaging relatives in the arrangement to go to clinic)
  - The Financial burden (Cost of travelling and doctor's fee)
  - The Emotional burden (Left stranded without medical advice in lockdown)

The overall resulting impact was a very satisfied patient the COVID-19 confinement situation

- **The Vision beyond the COVID-19 epidemic – The Growth of a Telemedicine Culture in society**

The learning that was necessary during COVID-19 introduced a culture of Telemedicine, making the implementation of Tele-OPD for chronic medical conditions such as Tele-dermatology, Tele-psychiatry, Tele-Rheumatology, Tele-cardiology and others very much easier than it had been in 2019. The lag to learning the concept of advanced Telemedicine systems such as Tele-Ward Round, Tele-Surgical Supervision, Tele-radiology, Tele-pathology and others was also reduced.

Summary of the widespread effect of Telemedicine

- Lowering the disease burden in the country
- Limiting the spread of COVID-19 infection in Pakistan
- Seeding a culture of Telemedicine within the public healthcare domain
- Lowering the barrier to adoption of Telemedicine by Doctors
- Setting a benchmark for the Healthcare Authorities
- Reducing the anxiety of Isolation and Social Circle regression
- Learning the Telemedicine Management Protocols as a new skill
- Realisation of the need for formal education in Telemedicine
- Serving as a Catalyst to several Telehealth projects in the country
- Triggering Entrepreneurship for Start-ups in Innovation in Telehealthcare

Governor & Chief Minister Punjab Telemedicine Helpline

Graphical Presentation of Tele-Consultations Data
13/05/2020 23:49

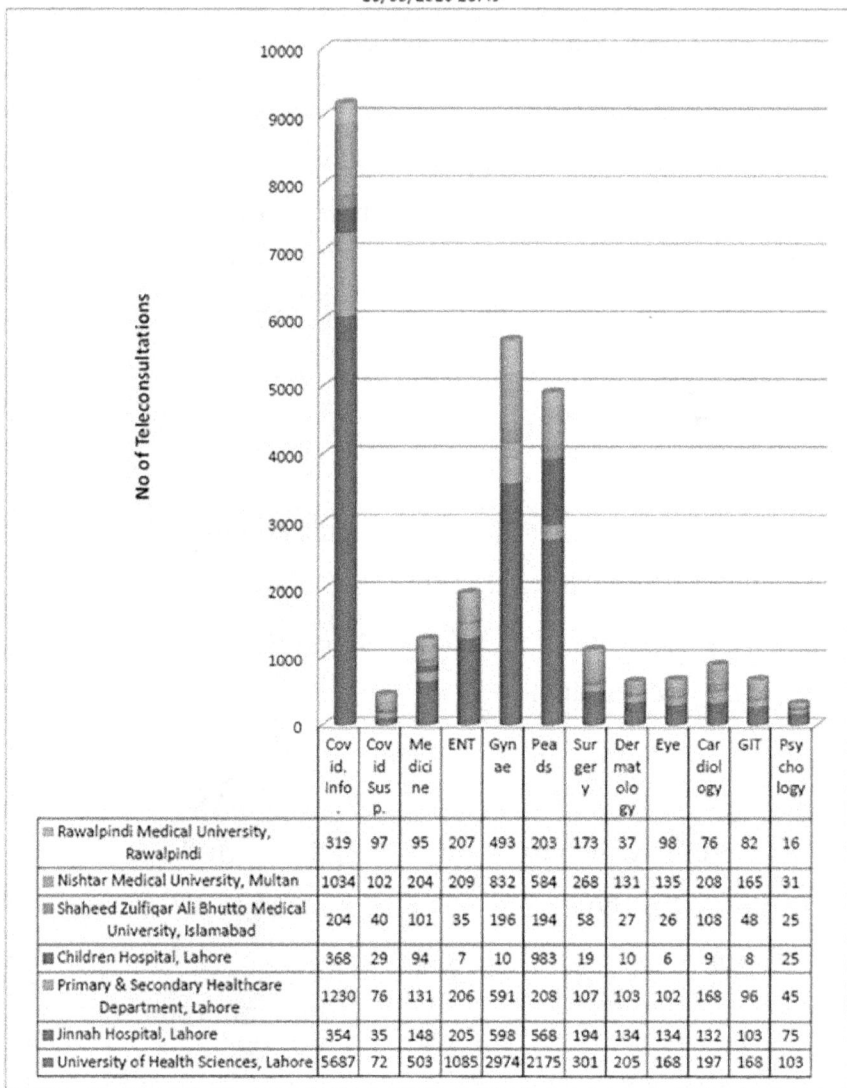

	Cov id. Info	Cov id Sus p.	Medicine	ENT	Gyn ae	Pea ds	Sur ger y	Der mat olo gy	Eye	Car diol ogy	GIT	Psy cho logy
Rawalpindi Medical University, Rawalpindi	319	97	95	207	493	203	173	37	98	76	82	16
Nishtar Medical University, Multan	1034	102	204	209	832	584	268	131	135	208	165	31
Shaheed Zulfiqar Ali Bhutto Medical University, Islamabad	204	40	101	35	196	194	58	27	26	108	48	25
Children Hospital, Lahore	368	29	94	7	10	983	19	10	6	9	8	25
Primary & Secondary Healthcare Department, Lahore	1230	76	131	206	591	208	107	103	102	168	96	45
Jinnah Hospital, Lahore	354	35	148	205	598	568	194	134	134	132	103	75
University of Health Sciences, Lahore	5687	72	503	1085	2974	2175	301	205	168	197	168	103

176

Governor & Chief Minister Punjab Telemedicine Helpline

Graphical Presentation of Tele-Consultations Data
16/05/2020 1:55

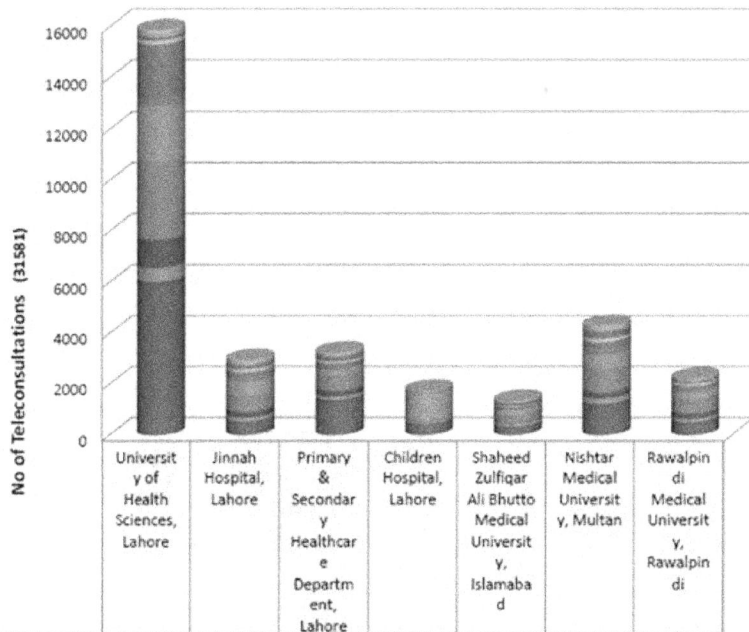

	University of Health Sciences, Lahore	Jinnah Hospital, Lahore	Primary & Secondary Healthcare Department, Lahore	Children Hospital, Lahore	Shaheed Zulfiqar Ali Bhutto Medical University, Islamabad	Nishtar Medical University, Multan	Rawalpindi Medical University, Rawalpindi
Psychology	107	76	51	25	27	51	21
GIT	171	121	106	14	61	194	91
Cardiology	104	145	179	11	117	241	81
Eye	189	140	109	14	41	161	109
Dermatology	2048	141	121	21	34	197	57
Surgery	322	201	109	20	61	281	184
Peads	2202	599	228	1057	245	609	284

177

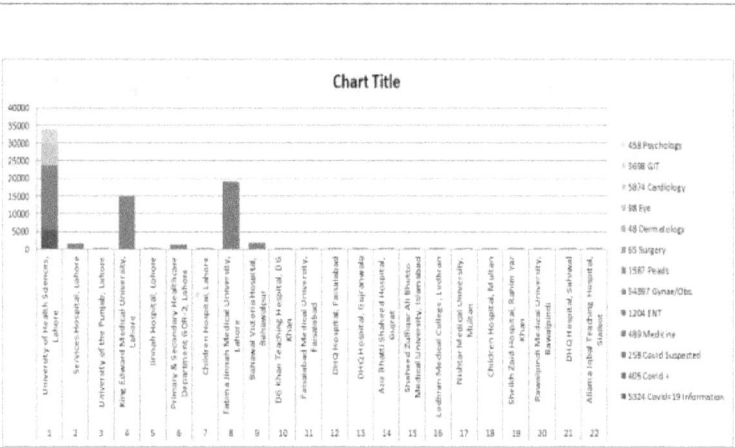

Chart Title

Legend:
- 458 Psychology
- 3698 GIT
- 5874 Cardiology
- 98 Eye
- 48 Dermatology
- 65 Surgery
- 1587 Peads
- 34397 Gynae/Obs.
- 1204 ENT
- 489 Medicine
- 259 Covid Suspected
- 405 Covid +
- 5324 Covid=19 Information

X-axis labels:
1. University of Health Sciences, Lahore
2. Services Hospital, Lahore
3. University of the Punjab, Lahore
4. King Edward Medical University, Lahore
5. Jinnah Hospital, Lahore
6. Primary & Secondary Healthcare Department, GOR-2, Lahore
7. Children Hospital, Lahore
8. Fatima Jinnah Medical University, Lahore
9. Bahawal Victoria Hospital, Bahawalpur
10. DG Khan Teaching Hospital, D.G. Khan
11. Faisalabad Medical University, Faisalabad
12. DHQ Hospital, Faisalabad
13. DHQ Hospital, Gujranwala
14. Aziz Bhatti Shaheed Hospital, Gujrat
15. Shaheed Zulfiqar Ali Bhutto Medical University, Islamabad
16. Lodhran Medical College, Lodhran
17. Nishtar Medical University, Multan
18. Children Hospital, Multan
19. Sheikh Zaid Hospital, Rahim Yar Khan
20. Rawalpindi Medical University, Rawalpindi
21. DHQ Hospital, Sahiwal
22. Allama Iqbal Teaching Hospital, Sialkot

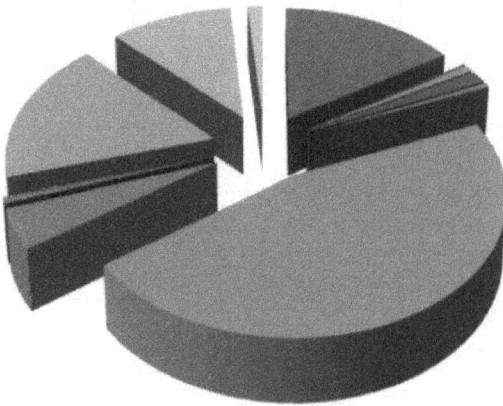

1 University of Health Sciences, Lahore

Legend:
- Covid=19 Information
- Covid +
- Covid Suspected
- Medicine
- ENT
- Gynae/Obs.
- Peads
- Surgery
- Dermatology
- Eye
- Cardiology
- GIT
- Psychology

125

Total No of Tele-Consultations (5,36,877)

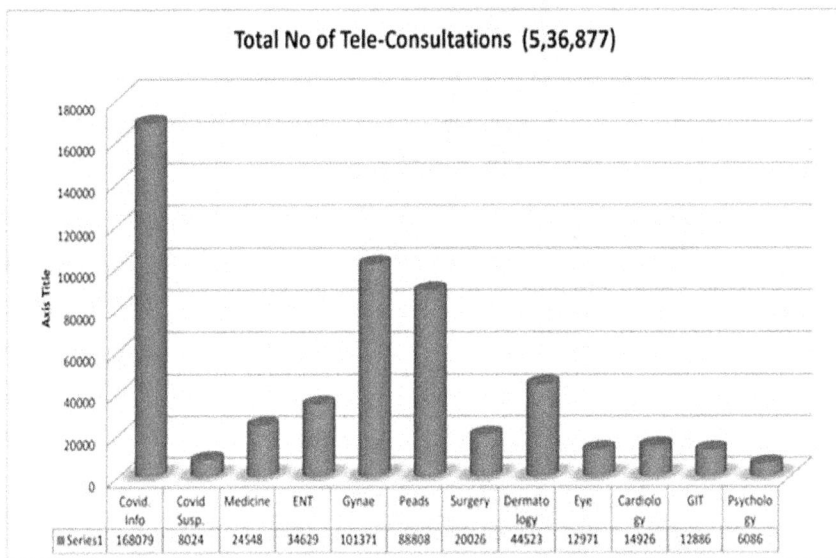

	Covid. Info	Covid Susp.	Medicine	ENT	Gynae	Peads	Surgery	Dermatology	Eye	Cardiology	GIT	Psychology
Series1	168079	8024	24548	34629	101371	88808	20026	44523	12971	14926	12886	6086

Chapter Ten

The Philosophy behind our Telemedicine Success

A "Bottom-Up" Management Process

Author: Prof W Angus Wallace
Co. Author: Dr Suhail Y Chughtai

Healthcare Management Challenges posed by the COVID-19 Pandemic

- Expected Crowding of Hospital Outpatients
- Doctors Falling Ill thus Resulting in Staff Shortages
- Shortage of Life Saving Equipment
- Limited Supply of COVID-19 Testing Kits
- Mental Strain of Isolation

Facilitation of Healthcare Services via Telemedicine in a Pandemic

- Availability of free medical advice at home 24/7
- Categorisation of patients
- Lowering the burden on Hospital Outpatient Departments
- Facilitation of Screening and Tracing
- Facilitation of Supply of Medications
- Relieving the mental strain

The Philosophy Behind our Telemedicine Success – Bottom-up management

The burgeoning adoption of Telemedicine and Telehealth services as an adjunct to the unprecedented COVID-19 pandemic has initiated dynamic and dramatic growth in remote healthcare delivery in Pakistan.

This growth is in response for the need to:

- provide needed access to clinicians for urgent and general requirements
- provide clinical protection to patients and providers to inhibit the spread of the virus
- advance the technology along with enhanced security concerns
- address regulatory and payment discrepancies that prohibit or limit service expansion; and address potential liability concerns.

Telemedicine and Telehealth being beneficial is clearly articulated by recent Centres of Disease Control COVID-19 guidance (June 10, 2020) (1)

- Screen patients who may have symptoms of COVID-19 and refer as appropriate
- Provide low-risk urgent care for non-COVID-19 conditions, identify those persons who may need additional medical consultation or assessment, and refer as appropriate

- Access primary care providers and specialists, including mental and behavioural health, for chronic health conditions and medication management
- Provide coaching and support for patients managing chronic health conditions, including weight management and nutrition counselling
- Participate in physical therapy, occupational therapy, and other modalities as a hybrid approach to in-person care for optimal health
- Monitor clinical signs of certain chronic medical conditions (e.g., blood pressure, blood glucose, other remote assessments)
- Engage in case management for patients who have difficulty accessing care (e.g., those who live in very rural settings, older adults, those with limited mobility)
- Follow up with patients after hospitalisation
- Deliver advance care planning and counselling to patients and caregivers to document preferences if a life-threatening event or medical crisis occurs
- Provide non-emergent care to residents in long-term care facilities
- Provide education and training for HCP through peer-to-peer professional medical consultations (inpatient or outpatient) that are not locally available, particularly in rural areas

Yet the regulatory and payment response, though rapid, requires a permanent solution. Issues surrounding payment inconsistency, state licensure and regulatory relief are discussed by Weigel et al. (2) that provides an essential overview of the regulatory opportunities and barriers. In an unpublished overview Farringer (3) provides an extensive historical perspective of the origins, regulatory waivers and changes and a prescription for future regulatory activities post COVID-19, that "improves coordination and cooperation" to remove barriers and enhance the quality of care and funding options.

Of course, the concerns relative to patient privacy, cybersecurity and consistent/reliable technological access are valid. It is incumbent on clinicians to adhere to both existing and temporary privacy protections. Patients who may have inadequate telephonic/internet access is a constant worry, particularly as related to illicit or unauthorised cyber security activities. The issue of clinical liability is a further concern, though insurance carriers are working to address the limitations of Telemedicine/Telehealth and adjusting coverage accordingly. (4)

The delivery of healthcare services has altered the clinical and business activities of physician practices and healthcare institutions. These entities have been faced with crisis management issues that many were unprepared to address. There has been a positive, and perhaps, permanent acceptance of Telemedicine and Telehealth that cannot be ignored.

The ability for clinicians to adapt to this new paradigm of clinical activity can only improve access to care, allow for improved coordination of care and provide for necessary regulatory and payment relief.

Reflections on our success six months later (in November 2020)

When Angus went into his self-imposed lockdown on 13th March 2020, he had already realised that the COVID-19 pandemic was going to create a crisis. It was a lucky coincidence that he had met with Professor Akram in London on 3rd March at the premises of Royal College of Physicians, London. The meeting proved to be vital because both Suhail and Angus had personal experience of using Telemedicine to manage patients. A plan to educate Pakistani doctors in Telehealth and Telemedicine was discussed to which Prof Akram was quite receptive.

The night before, after a private dinner at Suhail's home for Prof Akram and his wife Dr Shehla Javed along with some common friends, Suhail showed a practical demonstration of Telemedicine consultation in the home-set Telemedicine lab. Prof Akram appeared quite convinced of the usefulness of the technology. Angus provided Prof Akram with the reassurance that he had used Suhail's Telemedicine platform and had found it to be very functional.

This meeting of Angus and Suhail with Prof Akram appeared to have a bearing on the subsequent decision making by the authorities in Pakistan when Suhail proposed Telemedicine to be the solution of choice at a Press Conference on 12th March 2020 in Lahore for combating the menace of COVID-19 during the social distancing and lockdown phase.

The political will provided by the Governor of Punjab who worked in close liaison with Prof Akram, also the Vice-Chancellor of University of Health Sciences Lahore and what the country witnessed then turned out to be remote healthcare delivery revolution of significant scale.

Reflections on management systems

"Bottom-up" management occurs when goals, projects, and tasks are primarily informed by employee feedback. Employees are invited to participate in goal setting — sometimes simply with feedback, sometimes with a stake in the decision. The "bottom-up" management style isn't as readily used as top-down management is.

We believe that our progress with Telemedicine in Pakistan is a consequence of us being allowed to use a "bottom-up" management process effectively.

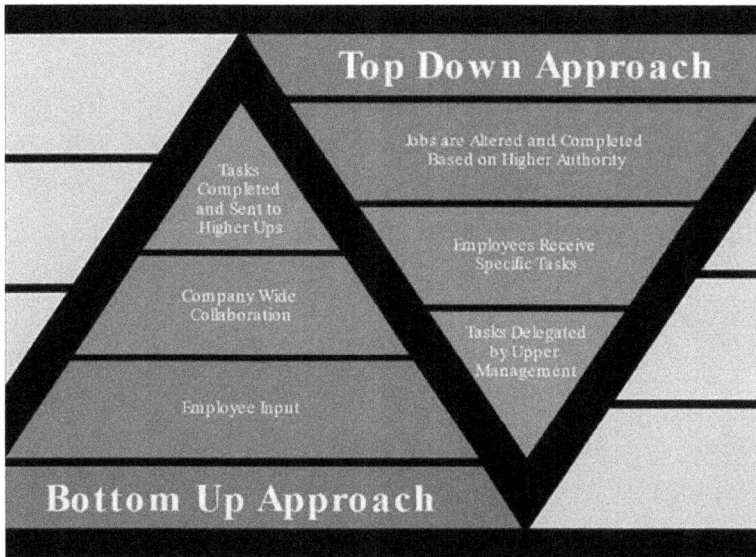

A "top-down" approach occurs where an executive decision-maker or other top person makes the decisions of how something should be done. This approach is disseminated under their authority to lower levels in the hierarchy, who are, to a greater or lesser extent, bound by them.

We believe that there can be severe problems with a "top-down" management system because those at the top may not be aware of what can be achieved and often recommend methods or processes that are not possible or practical. We, therefore, hope that many of those Telemedicine projects that are carried out in the future are processed with a "bottom-up" approach.

Our experience is that Telemedicine consultations at present are poorly understood and poorly implemented. Doctors and healthcare workers have not been trained to carry out an online consultation effectively, and many fail to appreciate how to modify their consultation techniques to make the patient more comfortable, in a way that can provide the maximum patient benefit.

The platform developed by Medical City Online is not only a high definition, secure and HIPAA compliant Video-consultation portal, but it also includes a complete appointment and practice management interface, seamlessly embedded into the system. Additionally, this particular software provides in-built Electronic Medical Records building up facility along with Prescription Writing facility. The features of this Telemedicine system by Medical City Online are detailed elsewhere in this book in a relevant chapter for the readers.

The information gathered can then be utilised via intelligent computer systems or Artificial Intelligence (AI) to provide the following:

- An audio recording of the consultation
- Automatic transcription of the audio recording into text
- Images of the patient (such as skin rashes, inspection of the mouth or ears, skin bruising, limb deformity or range of movement) providing visual documentation
- An auto-summary or the Consultation note that is created using AI
- Follow-up consultation appointments management facility
- Various medical measurements depending on digital equipment available – body temperature, pulse rate, blood pressure measurements, basic ECG recordings, blood oxygen (pO2) measurements, heart auscultation etc.
- Consent taking interface
- Facility for the patient to invite a family member into the virtual visit
- Facility for the doctor to invite a medical colleague into the consultation
- Facility for the Practice manager to invite an Interpreter into the consultation

We now believe that our COVID-19 pandemic has transformed the medical environment permanently and by using Telemedicine comprehensively, healthcare systems around the world can still deliver outpatient services remotely, with similar standards to those previously achieved with a face-to-face outpatient clinic appointment.

References

Services during the COVID-19 pandemic using Telehealth Services. CDC. gov June 10, 2020.

Weigal, Gabriela; Ramaswamy, Amrutha; Sobel, Laurie; Salganicoff, Alina; Cubanski Juliette; Freed, Meredith. Opportunities and Barriers for Telemedicine in the U.S. during the COVID-19 Emergency and Beyond. Kaiser Family Fund. May 11, 2020.

Farringer, Deborah. A Telehealth Explosion: Using Lessons from the Pandemic to Shape the Future of Telehealth Regulation. Texas A&M Law Review, Forthcoming Fall 2021. (Prepublication August 5, 2020).

Feldman, David L. How COVID-19 Accelerated Telemedicine Use. The Doctors Company and Health Risk Advisors. May 7, 2020.

Chapter Eleven

Interviews of Prof Dr Javed Akram & Dr Shehla Javed

Interviewers: Dr Fiona Hasan and Dr Ahmed Ijaz

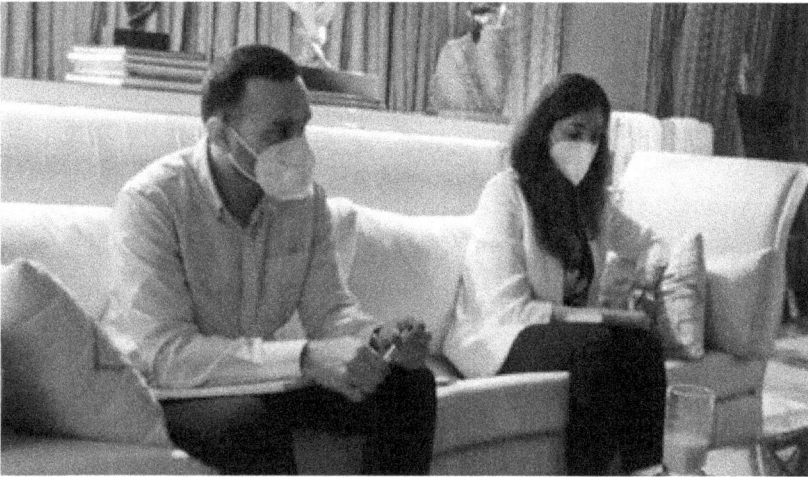

Prof Dr Javed Akram on Role of Telemedicine in Pakistan Healthcare

Question: Prof Dr Javed Akram, please tell us briefly about the current role in healthcare structure of Pakistan being a senior Clinician and Medical Educationist.

Answer: I am currently the Vice-Chancellor of University of Health Sciences, and also President Pakistan Society of Internal Medicine.

Question: How have you been associated with Telemedicine before the launch of the Helpline service?

Answer: We, in Pakistan, have been using various healthcare delivery systems for some 15 years, such as providing formal medical advice over telephone and using video cameras. We have also been using specialised Telemedicine services like telepathology and teleradiology by sending our radiographs and scanned images to other parts of the world to get a second opinion. Because the technology is becoming so common and relatively inexpensive, it is now within easy reach, thus more commonly available for medical professionals than before.

Question: How do you see Telemedicine facilitating healthcare delivery in Pakistan in the near future?

Answer: Telemedicine can be helpful for diagnostic Teleconsultations and then for treatment and then subsequent remote monitoring. Of course, Telemedicine is not supposed to be a replacement of a physical consultation because in Telemedicine, obviously the gentle touch, the hand-holding that patients expect cannot be provided. But short of that you can carry out most of the routine steps of a medical consultation with the modern Telemedicine technology.

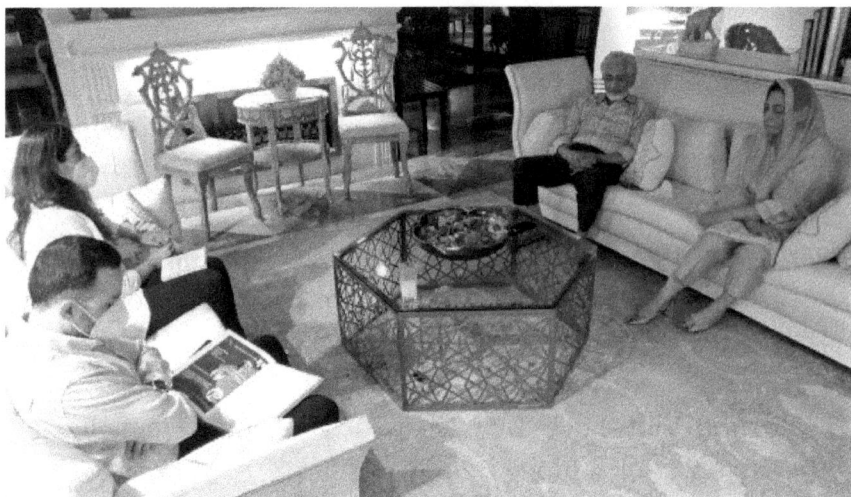

Question: How is Telemedicine shaping in Pakistan?

Answer: A common misperception is that "Telemedicine" is confused with "Teleconsultation" – they are not the same. Telemedicine is a clinician-patient encounter for which the most common means being adopted nowadays is a live two-way video which has brought a dynamic change into remote healthcare delivery. We often get images sent to us via WhatsApp to provide expert comments - this constitutes as a second opinion. In Telemedicine using the two-way live video, the patient can see you, your facial expressions and reactions on reading test results, etc. The facial gestures expressed through Telemedicine give a much better connection of the patients to the doctor, better than a telephonic consultation. The understanding of patients is on the rise and has been accelerated by the COVID-19 pandemic due to the necessitated use of Telemedicine services.

Question: How close is a virtual consultation with the doctor to a physical one?

Answer: In my view, Telemedicine is not just about taking the history of the patient. The video element of Telemedicine consultations established a two-way human communication bridge which helps to simulate it to become more like a physical meeting. A telephone or voice conversation alone does not produce the same effect. The visual examination replaces the conventional physical one, and certain adjustments have, therefore, to be made. The modern gadgets also provide remote cardiac auscultation through tele-stethoscopes. In the same way, remote ECG and Ultrasound transmission through the Telemedicine software is possible, which converts a virtual visit to look increasingly closer to a physical one.

For instance, looking inside the mouth for a throat examination, a closer and magnified look inside the ear and nose through Telemedicine cameras designed for the purpose are now widening the scope of remote healthcare delivery.

A doctor should know the limits of Telemedicine, and they are duty-bound to tell the patient when to ask for a physical consultation with the nearest available doctor if such a need arises. However, for repeat visits and basic health checks, where detailed physical examination is not obligatory or required, Telemedicine should eventually become the first choice as the care delivery tool.

In my view, the warmth of a physical consultation is not yet replaceable though for the sake of the patient's convenience or meeting certain conditions like the Corona pandemic, Telemedicine is the next best thing that has happened to the medical profession.

Question: Where do you see Telemedicine fit in "Fight against Corona Epidemic" as the Telemedicine Helpline Software designed by Dr Suhail Chughtai is helping a large number of patients with your University facilitating the project?

Answer: Of course, Telemedicine came to the rescue of all the physicians involved since COVID began to create havoc in this world. In Wuhan, China, since a doctor there was first diagnosed to have contracted the infection, it then spread rapidly all over the world.

We, in Pakistan, faced its first appearance in February and then it started becoming widespread in March 2020. We believe that because we deployed our Telemedicine facility, this helped us limit the spread alongside other measures taken by the government.

The timely deployment of the Telemedicine helpline, an idea that was shared at a press conference of the Pakistan Society of Internal Medicine 2020 by Dr Suhail Chughtai enabled a great self-defence mechanism. We found an alternative way of dealing with the pandemic, which was effective and within reach of common public confined at homes during the lockdown, which was announced in the middle of March 2020.

Question: Do you envisage Pakistan healthcare taking advantage of the advancements of Telemedicine systems?

Answer: Telemedicine has now become a little bit more advanced, particularly because many surgeons can now operate using Telemedicine, which we call Robotic Surgery. You can also carry out laser procedures on your eyes and operate through gloves with special controls operated remotely by a surgeon located elsewhere, such as remote robotic gastroscopy operations. The confidence of the public as consumers and doctors as providers has increased tremendously, which will pave the way for further evolution and development of the speciality Telemedicine sector, and this should be encouraged.

Question: Do you have any plans to introduce formal education in Telemedicine at your University of Health Sciences, Pakistan?

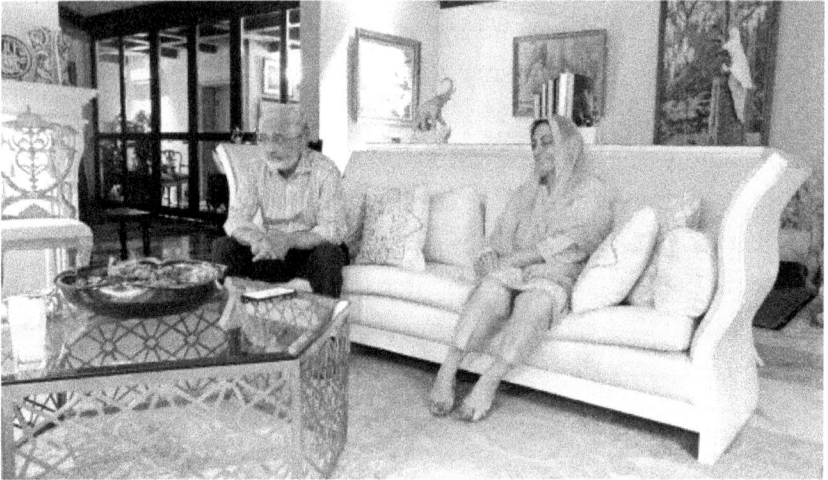

Answer: So, we at our University of Health Sciences (UHS, Lahore) thought, why not create Telemedicine specialists? Doctors like me were a bit familiar with the technology. But if you want to teach it as a subject, then you need a specialist who can teach our undergraduates and postgraduates. All Telemedicine applications, whether invasive or non-invasive or just observation or advancing this technology, need trained users and teachers. So we thought we would encourage people to take it up as a speciality. That is why we have started our six-month diploma course for training in Telemedicine, and to include its application in different specialities such as cardiology, gynaecology, dermatology, etc.

We need to go further than the deployment of Telemedicine systems in the country. We need to have a diploma qualification in Telemedicine, progressing to a master's degree and PhD. It was my idea of having this diploma in Telemedicine as one module of the master's degree program in Health Informatics, Telehealth and Artificial Intelligence. So, a four-month module training in Telemedicine has now been set up. Another module is the Hospital Information Management System, HIMS.

The third module is public health informatics, the outbreak, in other words, epidemics, hotspots, predicting which disease is going to come next, and how prevalent it is likely to be.

That is really public health digitisation, and then the fourth is the software development within the health framework. You develop your own practice software, you modify the software which is available to you, just for basic programming. And then the last thing is that these can benefit students who will be taking this up as a career, they will have to work for three months in a digital hospital. We have already identified the faculty of local and international experts which is being created. So that is why doctors or nurses or paramedics need to become very familiar with technology on the digital side.

Question: Coming back to the Telemedicine Helpline at Doctors 24/7 Online website project, created back in March. How do you see the journey from that point on? And what was the biggest challenge you faced in the setting?

Answer: The project was challenging, mainly because we were not prepared for it, even the world was not prepared for it. For those who travelled internationally, there was panic. And then, of course, the worst thing is that it carries a mortality of up to 2%. With this level of mortality, even the developed world struggled with it and are still struggling. So, anything related to COVID was very challenging, and no institution had developed any plans for it.

The Outpatient departments of the hospitals across Pakistan were getting crowded. And in hospitals like General Hospital, they had about 9000 plus patients coming in every day for a check-up, travelling hundreds of miles just to get seen by specialists for ruling out Coronavirus. As the hospital outpatient departments closed, 9000 people every day were denied consultation.

As they could not afford access to private healthcare, the chaos started building up as these patients would die without any medical help. The biggest challenge was to create an alternative pathway for them. They were suffering from diabetes, hypertension, stroke, heart conditions. Another challenge was lack of familiarity of patients with computers, software or mobile apps because a large proportion of the population belongs to a humble socioeconomic background.

Question: Apart from logistic issues, what other barrier had to be lifted to make Telemedicine take off in Pakistan at community care level?

Answer: Raising awareness about the benefits of the Telemedicine service was needed. We were also aware that 23% of Pakistan has no connectivity for 3G or Wi-Fi.

Now, even if there was connectivity, a significant proportion of the people did not have smartphones or tablets, including a small proportion of our medical students.

Question: Do you see Telemedicine use in Pakistan continue beyond the COVID-19 pandemic?

Answer: The confidence gained by patients using Telemedicine during the lockdown is helping the industry grow in Pakistan. With an increasing number of Telemedicine providers in the country, the options available for the consumer (patient) and provider (doctor) have made life easier for both. It is a natural evolution of the industry where we can be seen to be making progress in General Telemedicine, and we are also now beginning to touch specialised Telemedicine, such as teledermatology, telecardiology, etc.

The computers, webcams and internet bandwidth are within affordable reach of doctors and the urban population, while those who cannot afford a computer can still use a smartphone and carry out online consultation using their local network bandwidth or domestic Wi-Fi connection.

I am hopeful that young physicians using our Telemedicine service will inspire a senior generation while the atmosphere is becoming more and more conducive for this game-changing method of healthcare delivery.

One of the most significant motives for Telemedicine in Pakistan to become popular is in order to create a bridge between a Basic Health Unit in a rural or suburban area and a District or Tehsil Headquarter Hospital.

The COVID-19 pandemic has revolutionised care delivery, and we now see ourselves in a position to deploy measures like Telemedicine Centres within a short time. Given the political will shown by the Governor of Punjab, I was able to back up the creation of the Telemedicine Helpline at the University of Health Sciences within 48 hours, after which the Governor was invited to launch the service on 18th March.

Question: How did you motivate the medical professionals to take part in Doctors 24/7 Telemedicine Helpline Project as there was no financial reward?

Answer: The specialist consultants and young doctors were supported very well. Without them, the materialisation of this project would never have been possible. They were the main soldiers, our front-line soldiers in the fight against Covid who worked 24/7 to provide free medical advice on *www.Doctor247.online* backed up by our telephone lines. We arranged their pickup and drop, food and a comfortable work environment. We also promised to provide them with certificates to acknowledge their voluntary service.

They were trained by Dr Suhail Chughtai on his designed Telemedicine website with the local UHS team on ground to take care of the ground operations. The young doctors who registered in large numbers (over 500) were managed by the operations team for the process of selection, training, and quality control.

Dr Shehla Javed on Women Entrepreneurship in Telemedicine Sector

Question: Dr Shehla Javed, please give us a brief about your roles and responsibilities.

Answer: I am Dr Shehla Javed and I practice as a consultant nutritionist in Lahore. I am also the founder and former chairperson of the Women Chamber of Commerce and Industry in Pakistan. Besides my clinical practice, I also manage my own business, a pharmaceutical company in Lahore.

Question: What is your take on women entrepreneurship in the sector of growing Telemedicine industry in Pakistan?

Answer: I promote women for businesses and encourage them to take up entrepreneurial roles. Given the new situation faced due to COVID-19, we felt ready to face it using Telemedicine as a tool at my private hospital setup. A few months before the Covid pandemic, I had decided to introduce Telemedicine at my private hospital, and the service was in the process of being set up when we were struck by the Covid pandemic which changed a lot of things as people developed a fear of coming to the hospital, both in private and public sector, to avoid the risk of contracting COVID-19 from the expanding pandemic in Pakistan.

Telemedicine came to the rescue and connected people back to their carers through a noticeable proportion of patients have sensitive cultural norms and needed to see the doctor while keeping their head covered.

We received feedback that female patients worry about the risk of recording the video conversation off the screen or even taking pictures of the screen during the examination which at times requires exposure of some part of the body. A woman visiting a doctor in person would know the situation in the examination room, but during a Telemedicine consultation, the female patients were never sure of who else was behind the camera or in the room watching the screen. This provoked a sense of reluctance within a sector of female patients who turned away from the use of Telemedicine.

This feedback within 3 to 4 weeks of the helpline service made us think, and then I suggested the idea of a "Pink Telemedicine" service where the examining doctor would be female for a female patient.

Such a service would give the female patient confidence to talk openly and allow her to show parts of the body which she would otherwise be shy or reluctant to show on the grounds of secrecy. A special icon which, if clicked, would bring a female patient to the online clinic of an online female doctor was created and thus our problem was solved.

Such a service was easy to set up with the Doctors 24/7 Online web administrator making some quick adjustments, while the female doctor's roster was amended to provide round the clock cover. Transport arrangements for pickup and drop of female doctors were made from various centres especially at the University of Health Sciences to ensure comfort and safety for all the health workers working at late hours of the night or early hours of the morning.

Pink Telemedicine addressed the fears of our female patients in the general public using our Telemedicine service and helped promote the concept of Telemedicine Helpline.

Question: Is your strategy of bringing women into the digital health space working towards success?

Answer: Women in business in Pakistan would benefit enormously from support coming from like-minded women who have the capability of creating opportunities. Through my experience of managing the Women's Chamber of Commerce and Industry Pakistan, I felt confident in raising entrepreneurship opportunities for women in the country who wanted to thrive in business and for this matter, in the Telemedicine industry.

Mrs Governor Punjab showed her interest in being a part of such a drive by joining us. Later I was joined by the PPIF (Punjab Population Innovation Fund) team who work on outreach programs. I supported the idea and spoke to the Telemedicine Helpline administration to develop an understanding and collaboration between the Telemedicine Helpline administration, the Women's Chamber of Commerce and Industry Pakistan, PPIF and the Sarwar Foundation headed by Mrs Governor Punjab.

The Telemedicine Helpline administration worked well with the idea of Pink Telemedicine and also with the advantage of a call analysis and data review (designed by the Helpline Administration). We were in a better position to suggest to the government that we should place our emphasis on the right sectors of disease burden such as mother and child issues of specific nature, mental health issues of women confined in lockdown, etc.

Question: How far you think your initiative will go beyond COVID-19?

Answer: I thought that Pink Telemedicine provided a good window to study the specifics of disease burden in women and child health diseases. The analytical review of the data acquired helped us understand the direction in which funds should be spent while setting priorities for managing diseases in the community.

Pink Telemedicine opened a thought window where women can control the choices suitable for preserving their privacy while benefiting from the advanced technology of remote care, where cultural values could be a barrier to the propagation of the service.

I also believe that the propagation of Telemedicine will help reduce and abolish quackery which is a stigma of the medical profession. If a member of the public knows that a doctor is available in a remote village over Telemedicine, he or she is likely to avoid seeing a non-medical practising person who is playing with the ignorance of the underprivileged community.

Prof Dr Javed Akram

FRCP (Ed. Glasgow), FACP (USA), FACC (USA)
FASIM (USA), M.D

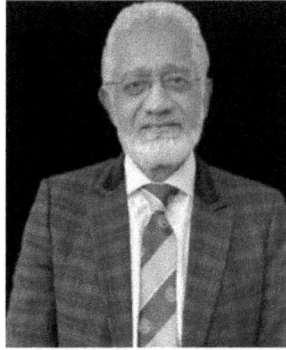

- Vice-Chancellor of University of Health Sciences, Pakistan (current)
- Shaheed Zulfiqar Ali Bhutto Medical University as Vice-Chancellor
- Pakistan Institute of Medical Sciences, (PIMS), Islamabad as CEO
- Medical Education to Government of Punjab as Advisor
- Head of Department of Medicine, Jinnah Hospital, Lahore
- Allama Iqbal Medical College, Lahore as Chairman Academic Council
- Allama Iqbal Medical College Lahore as Principal
- Jinnah Hospital Lahore as Chief Executive Officer
- King Edward Medical College/ University, Lahore as Head of Department of Medicine

Prof Dr Javed Akram has specialised in Internal Medicine and has special expertise in managing and treating Diabetes. Prof Akram has an illustrious career in medical teaching and research, drawing respect from all sectors of the healthcare profession in and out of Pakistan.

He is the President of the Pakistan Society of Internal Medicine, a prominent medical organisation with multi-city Chapters in Pakistan.

Prof Akram has been awarded several awards including, National Award for contribution in the field of medical education awarded by the Government of Pakistan, Tamgha-e-Imtiaz (Pride of Performance) by the Government of Pakistan on 23rd March 2012, Chief Minister Punjab's Gold Medal in 2010 in recognition of his outstanding services for the well-being of ailing humanity.

Dr Shehla Javed

Founder President at Women Chamber of Commerce and Industry, Pakistan

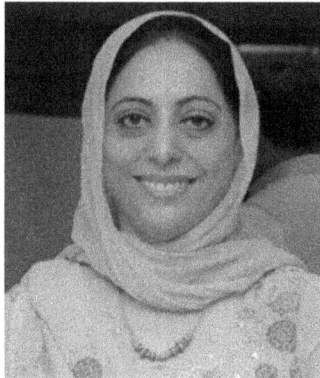

Dr Shehla Javed Akram is one of the successful women entrepreneurs in Pakistan and has more than half a dozen companies to her name. She became a pioneer in the field of healthcare when she and her husband launched Pakistan's first hospital for acute medical care. She then broke into the traditionally male-dominated pharmaceutical sector by setting up a pharmaceutical business. Most recently, she became the CEO of a real estate development company, JS Developers.

In the public sector, Dr Shehla struggled for seven years to get approval for establishing a separate Women's Chamber of Commerce and Industry in Pakistan. This innovative idea occurred after she won the election as an executive member in the LCCI election on open merit in the year 2002 and became the first woman Executive Committee member of the Lahore Chamber of Commerce and Industry, after realising that women entrepreneurs cannot excel in a male dominant chamber mainly because of their own inhibitions and that women-specific products needed a more dedicated platform. Finally, the national assembly passed the bill for addition in SRO to allow Women Chambers at provincial/ divisional/district levels and thus she became the founder president of the Women's Chamber of Commerce and Industry in Pakistan.

As a result, from a single seat representation in 2002, it has increased by 172% to date with one seat reserved for the vice-president FPCCI from the Women's Chamber of Commerce and Industry. This increased representation has also encouraged policymakers to define better gender-specific policies to encourage women in the Small and Medium sized Enterprise (SME) sector along with improved legislation for the status of women.

Under her leadership the Women's Chamber of Commerce and Industry has become an internationally recognised forum with ECOSOC, working actively for the promotion of women entrepreneurship in Pakistan. She became the First Vice-President of the Federation of Pakistan Chambers of Commerce and Industry. She also sits on the Board of Directors of PAMCO, SDC Punjab, Member Board of Governor PMEIF, and Ambassador for International Women (OPS).

Chapter Twelve

The Way Forward - Telemedicine to Revolutionise Healthcare

Healthcare Administration in Pakistan to incorporate Telemedicine

Author: Captain(R) Muhammad Usman (Provincial Health Secretary, Punjab)

Preface of Telemedicine Project

The Primary and Secondary Healthcare Department, Punjab took revolutionary steps towards curtailing the COVID-19 emergency while establishing a strong, sustainable, and integrated Healthcare System in the most populated province of the country. Punjab saw a slow increase in positivity during the first few months of the pandemic.

The first case was reported in March 2020, but the peak was reached at the beginning of June 2020. The initial reduction in positive cases was reached through a number of administrative actions taken to avoid the projected trend of high death rate and positivity. These include aggressive contact tracing, increased testing, compulsory quarantine of 100% confirmed cases in government facilities or public/ private hospitals and massive awareness drives for the public.

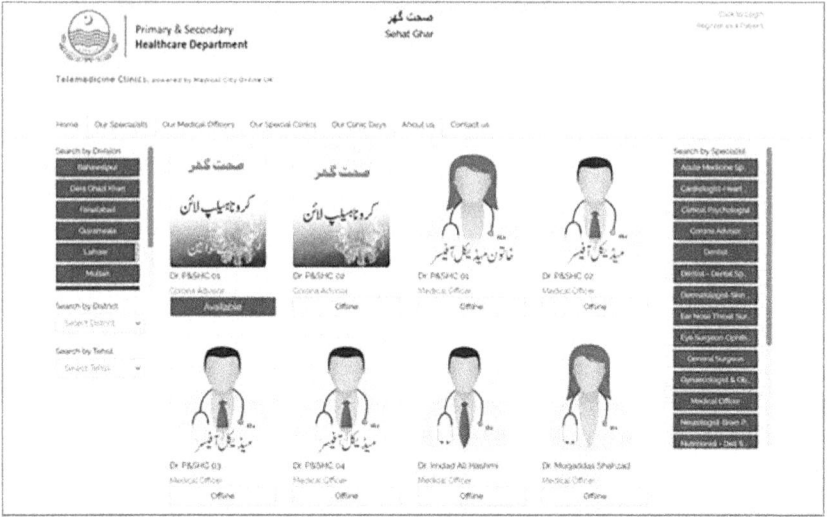

Side by side, owing to the continuous threat and continuous prevalence of the virus, Primary & Secondary Healthcare Department launched a synchronised and structured Telemedicine pilot project. The revolutionary initiative of Telemedicine emphasises reducing the burden of both COVID-19 and non-COVID diseases during the pandemic of COVID-19, on healthcare facilities also building

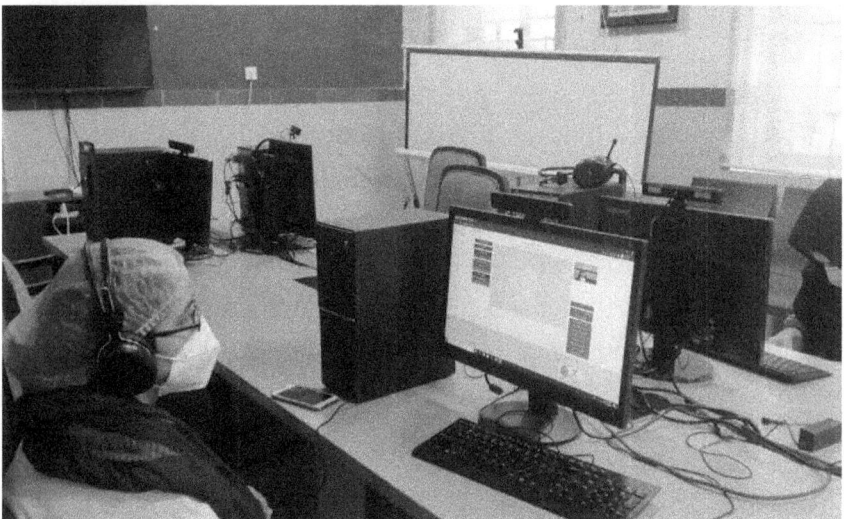

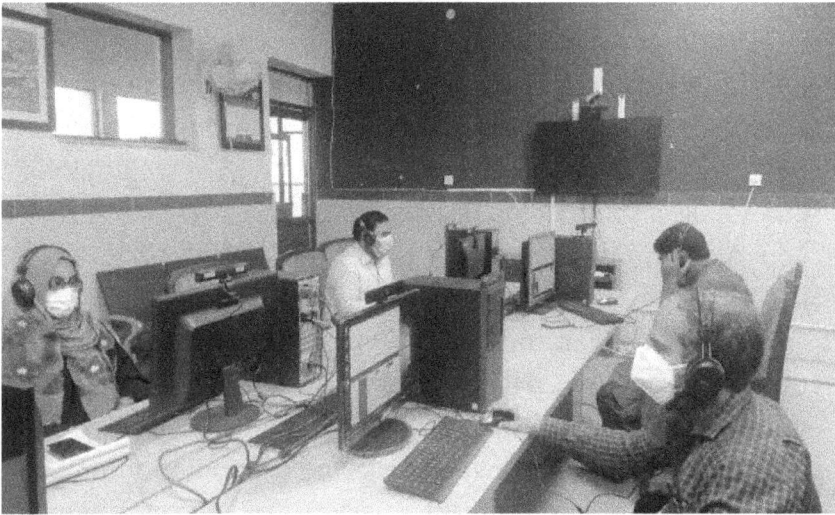

public confidence on an alternative mode of information. This initiative was built around developing connectivity across various health facilities in rural and urban areas without requiring patient movement to tertiary care hospitals unless required for treatment.

The Pakistan Telemedicine initiative is beginning to virtually transform the communication and clinical diagnosis rendered under the existing healthcare system to ensure the continued provision of medical consultation services even in the worsening situation of COVID-19.

This Telemedicine initiative is not only going to reduce the burden on Government hospitals but is also helping to organise the triage of healthcare system in concordance with EMR. Telemedicine is improving documentation in such a way that all clinical data on an individual basis becomes traceable, utilisable, audit-able and brings benefit and ease for patients, clinicians, healthcare providers, public health specialists and Government for policy making.

The ambition behind this program was to develop an integrated and consolidated healthcare system "Sehat Aap Ke Ghar Tak" or Health at Your Doorstep encompassing all Health Facilities and Vertical Programs through advanced EMR and Telemedicine to promote healthcare facilities for accessible and efficient healthcare services in both urban and rural areas. Connecting patients visiting at the Basic Health Units across the nine Divisions of Punjab with the specialists at Tehsil and District Headquarters through Sehat Ghar (Telemedicine project) is a mission being achieved and once accomplished, this will be Pakistan's largest virtual healthcare delivery network covering a population of 110 million people, a significant mission and a dream worth giving best efforts for.

The primary focus is on the provision of specialised consultations to the periphery population, thus playing a vital role in improving access to healthcare, reducing geographic barriers, and optimising healthcare for patients.

In the second phase of the project, incorporation of pharmacies, laboratory services and blood testing services will be included so that patients can get complete home-based healthcare services where objectively possible.

Captain(R) Muhammad Usman Younis
Secretary of Health, Punjab, Pakistan

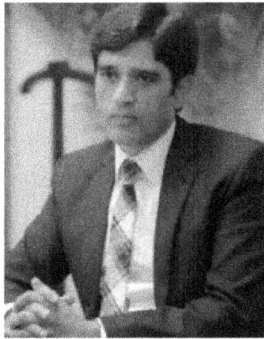

Civil Servant (BS-20)
Pakistan Administrative Service

* Deputy Commissioner Astore
* Deputy Commissioner Gilgit
* Home Secretary, Gilgit
* Secretary Punjab Workers Welfare Board, Punjab
* District Coordination Officer, Rajanpur, Punjab
* Additional Director General, Parks & Horticulture Authority, Lahore, Punjab
* Cane Commissioner, Punjab
* Director Food District Coordination Officer/Deputy Commissioner, Lahore
* Director General, Punjab Food Authority
* Secretary, Primary & Secondary Healthcare, Government of Punjab

Captain (R) Muhammad Usman Younis joined the Pakistan Administrative Service in the year 2000 before serving in uniform for nine years.

He has served in Punjab, Sindh and Gilgit Baltistan. He has held important and impactful positions during the last 29 years of service.

Captain (R) Usman has championed the cause of Public Health throughout his career as during his tenure as District Coordination Officer, Lahore he successfully managed the Dengue epidemic in 2014, 2015 and 2016. His effective leadership for field teams during Polio drives was remarkable, leading to Lahore being Polio free during his tenure. Under his leadership, the dengue epidemic of 2019 in Rawalpindi was controlled in time which otherwise could have resulted in a potentially bigger disaster. The timely actions taken during his posting as Secretary Primary and Secondary Healthcare Department were instrumental in averting a major health disaster.

The COVID-19 pandemic exposed the current health infrastructure to many unforeseen challenges globally as well as within Punjab. Captain (R) Usman took on the challenge and demonstrated exceptional leadership skills engaging all stakeholders as early as January 2020. He envisaged and utilised the Technical Working Group to author over 20 Standard Operating Procedures for different levels and target audience to give easy to understand protocols and guidelines to follow.

From zero testing ability in February 2020 to testing capability of over 18,000 tests/day in June, he developed and laid down a comprehensive laboratory network system that catered to populations across Punjab. He visited each laboratory and assessed the quality of work and instructed on changes that could be made for optimal utilisation. His visionary steps allowed the department and the government to respond to the health emergency at hand and have validated data for early case response. The Punjab COVID-19 Reporting MIS data was developed to ensure live reporting of cases from all public and private sector laboratories and case management in public and private hospitals to provide a holistic review of the situation on ground and plan accordingly.

Under his supervision, a comprehensive Health Management system was launched with an Integrated COVID-19 Reporting MIS to collect data from all public and private health sector hospitals and laboratories for up-to-date situation reporting. Side by side, a Laboratory MIS was developed to provide real-time result to all potential and confirmed cases being tested in Public and Private sector labs. The sample management was improved with unique identifications being given to individual samples to provide traceability.

The healthcare providers were amply looked after with the development of a Resource Management System to give ground details of provision and stock inventory of PPEs at each health facility. First responders were equipped through a separate application with a detailed health facility wise ventilator vacancy position to make informed decisions about where to take critical patients. Captain (R) Usman also established a Contact Tracing Unit at the provincial level which monitored all field formations on contact tracing, and which has resulted in over 600,000 contacts being traced and tested. Punjab has seen a steady decline in positivity from over 40% to below 2% within five months.

Chapter Thirteen

Evolution of Telemedicine in Pakistan

History of Growth and Evolution

Author: **Mr Saflain Haider**

Context

Pakistan's total population is 204,774,520 million, with an urban population of just over 39%. The primary infrastructure of the country spans over 5,000 Basic Health Units (BHUs), 600 Rural Health Centres (RHCs), 7500 other first-level care facilities and over 100,000 lady health workers.

On average, a village in rural Punjab is located 8 kilometres away from the nearest BHU. Moreover, 20% of the rural population do not have a BHU within 10 kilometres of the village, while 22% of them do not have RHC within 10 kilometres of the village.

The figure shows geographical dispersion of BHUs and RHCs across Punjab. Red and green coloured icons depict BHUs and RHCs, respectively.

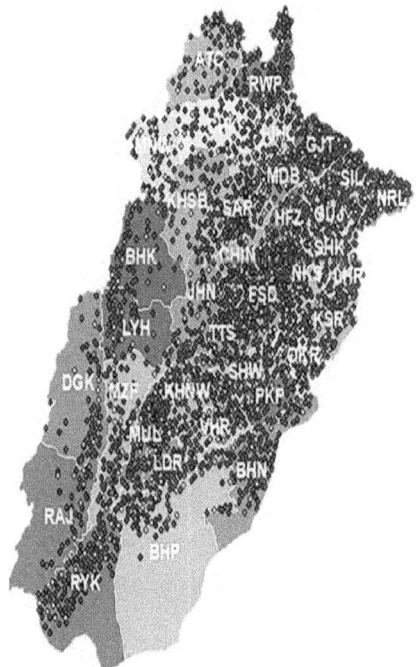

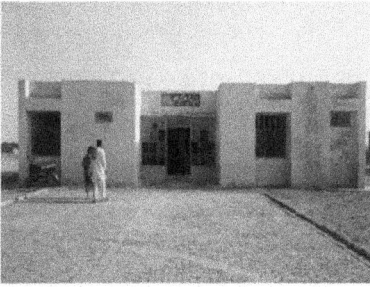
BHU Dragal
Power Outage

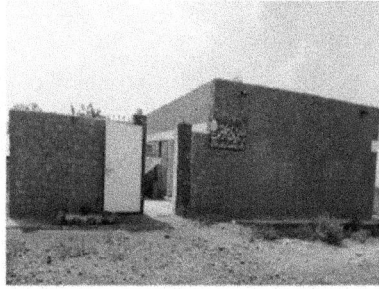
BHU Nari
Doctor's Non availability

The global standard mandates the availability of two doctors, a dentist and eight nurses for around 1,000 people are needed to provide adequate coverage with primary care interventions. The number of primary healthcare facilities isn't enough to cater to the health needs of the population. The acute shortage of doctors has risen to 0.4 million, where we need 1.6 million nurses to meet international standards. Pakistan being the sixth most populous country of the world operates healthcare systems which date back to medieval.

It is relatively common to find primary facilities where posts of dedicated doctors are vacant. This relates to a problem where Pakistan faces a sheer shortage of qualified doctors resulting due to brain drain. According to an estimate, almost 70% of medical students in colleges/ universities are female, and a significant percentage of them do not pursue the medical profession after marriage barring cultural challenges. Placement of doctors on a permanent basis in primary healthcare facilities stays a priority for governments in Pakistan whereby remote area allowances are introduced, and service in primary healthcare facilities have been assigned specific percentage in central induction policy (CIP).

Recent amendments in the constitution of Pakistan has mandated devolution in the healthcare sector; provinces use policies which are neither uniform nor target collective goal to improve on service delivery KPIs for the entire country. Khyber Pakhtunkhwa (North-Western Province of Pakistan) introduced a policy where purpose-built dorms are made with provisioning of complimentary transportation services to doctors appointed in remote areas. Government of Punjab has upgraded more than 1200 primary healthcare facilities lately in terms of general outlook, availability of services, presence of doctors and paramedical staff and hours of operations. The added feature list includes pickup services for pregnant mothers and transfer of complicated cases to secondary and tertiary healthcare facilities.

Provincial governments are committed to uplift service delivery by resolving challenges related to medicine availability, doctor's placements, cleanliness, availability of trained medical skilled workers and provisioning of utilities. Let alone the effectiveness of government-owned primary healthcare facilities, assuming the primary sector magically starts performing at par; Pakistan still faces an issue in terms of coverage. The inefficiency of the primary healthcare regime creates an unnecessary burden on tertiary and secondary care facilities located in the major cities.

Needless to say, this leads to compromised care delivery, healthcare regime once rated best in the region is going down drastically. Primary care setup of our country is neither efficient nor provides **outreach to locations where it matters the most.** The financial crunch does not present the freedom to set up new brick and mortar structures throughout the country and especially when even existing facilities are not managed in the most optimum fashion.

The situation is no different in government-owned secondary and tertiary healthcare facilities where availability of consultants (paediatrician, neurologist, gastrologist and other specialities) is a challenge.

Tech Centric Solutions

Traditionally, the placement of doctors in remote areas has been a challenge. Governments have tried various models such as topping up monthly salary with placement allowances. The model initially rated as success seems like a failure now as sustainable placement is becoming an issue.

Clustering Model

In 2017, the Primary and Secondary Healthcare Department (P&SH) identified 50 BHUs in four districts of Punjab, where traditionally doctor availability had been an issue. The model categorised two neighbouring BHUs as a single cluster where the doctor was asked to be physically present in each BHU on alternate days. The patients from the facility where the doctor wasn't present that day were seen remotely using classic Telemedicine.

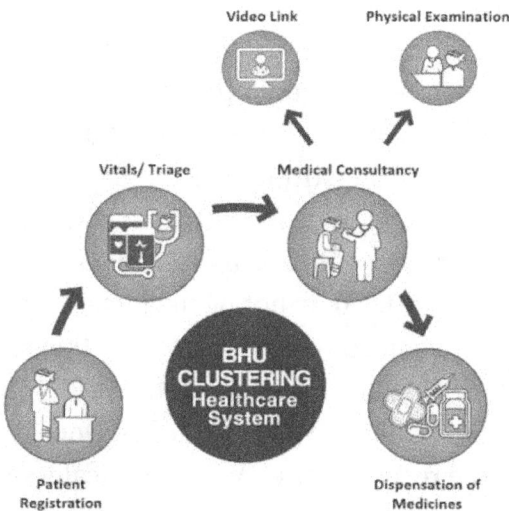

Video Link　　　Physical Examination

Vitals/ Triage　　Medical Consultancy

BHU CLUSTERING Healthcare System

Patient Registration　　　Dispensation of Medicines

Punjab Information Technology Board (PITB), the implementation partner for P&SH implemented the entire care delivery protocol while deploying the Telemedicine solution. This included registration of patients, capturing of vitals, physical/remote consultation and dispensation of medicine. The tech didn't only help ensure provisioning of consultations but digitised the patient experience throughout the interaction.

Selected BHUs typically reported daily patient count of 25 (non-verifiable) which sky-rocketed to as many as 70 after deployment of Telemedicine. Authorities also used contact information of the patient to fire an automated SMS questionnaire to enquire about the standard of service delivery and dispensation of free medicine. Software solution based on WebRTC was used to facilitate Telemedicine. Three computers/laptops were handed over to each BHU dedicated for registration counter/vitals station, doctor consultation room and medicine dispensation room. Supported through dedicated training sessions, the system was up and running within a few months.

One Hub to Many

Typically, provincial setups in entire Pakistan are focussed on placing doctors in primary healthcare facilities, which seems like the best possible solution as any other medium may not substitute the presence of a physical doctor. Keeping in view the overall shortage of doctor and limitations of forcing a doctor to stay in an area deprived of even basic necessities may not be neglected. It was shocking to learn during inspection visits that expecting mothers were comfortable seeing Lady Health Visitor (LHV) than deputed Woman Medical Officer (WMO, Qualified Doctor). Curious as we all were the response was "WMOs typically serve in BHUs for few months only whereas LHVs are always here so we might as well see her for consultation".

Even 95% of doctor's placement on an official document in the government department present an opposite picture in reality. Primary and Secondary Healthcare Department in late 2017 envisioned a project where 250 BHUs were to be connected with the central hub of doctors. The pilot runs limited to four BHUs registered staggering 25,000 patients in a period of four months. With more than 18,000 remote consultations, the initiative revolutionised the entire healthcare regime where a referral system was launched as a by-product to refer patients to secondary healthcare facilities of the district.

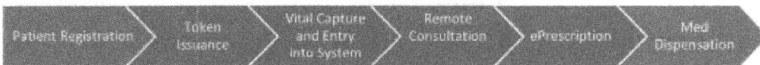

Patient Registration > Token Issuance > Vital Capture and Entry into System > Remote Consultation > ePrescription > Med Dispensation

The initiative mandated an availability of qualified Assistant Clinical Analyst with a know-how of basic ICT to capture vital statistics and enter these into the system, establish a connection with the doctor and printing the prescription written by the doctor remotely. Third world countries struggle with the availability of motivated and dedicated workforce, especially in the government sector, therefore services of Asst. Clinical Analyst was outsourced to the private sector.

The initiative gained recognition within no time, and the BHUs were named eBHUs where not only daily patient count whizzed, but patients were coming back after the treatment saying, "We wanted to thank the doctor for the treatment".

Typical consultation cost to government if the physical doctor is available in BHU is estimated at $1.19, which reduces to $0.71 if the doctor is available in a central hub and provides consultation remotely. With a shortage of doctors throughout the country, placing a dedicated doctor in BHU may not be practical. The model enables authorities to depute one doctor to cater to a patient load of 1.5 BHUs.

Specialised Consultations

The model has been in use in Pakistan for a decade, but the last few years have witnessed its implementations in a wide array of areas by various entities. Government of Punjab through its tech partner, PITB implemented various initiatives where BHUS of DG Khan division were connected with notable tertiary hospitals of the provincial capital. One such model connects Service Hospital for Nephrology and Neurology and Children Hospital for Paediatrics and Pead Cardiology. Reaching out to BHUs in remotest areas, internet availability presented challenges for which satellite connectivity has been used where deemed necessary. As expensive as it may sound in the past, occasional linkages using this medium are pretty much possible when it comes to saving the lives of thousands. Digital probes are also provided wherever necessary to facilitate Medical Officers in clinical assessment and onward submission to specialists.

Probes on Rotation

Sub-National Governance (SNG) Program in Pakistan implemented a pilot project in District Sheikhupura where ultrasound devices and other necessary equipment were handed over to the private sector and a cluster of six nearing BHUs were identified. The team would share a plan in advance to be available at each facility on each day of the week. Patients would turn up, and the female technician would assist in ultrasound. Gynaecologist sitting on the other side would see the images in real-time and provide consultation.

The system is appreciated at all forums, and there are plans to expand its implementation in other districts.

COVID-19 and Telemedicine

The Recent pandemic of COVID-19 has brought the entire world to a halt. As of 16th November 2020, the world has witnessed as many as 54.3 million reported cases of COVID-19 with the number of tragic deaths over 1.3 million. When it comes to leading the life in a pandemic, more than anybody else, patients struggled and feared to visit hospitals as countries were forcing lockdowns. Humongous population with already overstretched and compromised health delivery network, Pakistanis had fewer options to consider. Rising to the occasion Tech came to rescue in connecting people with sane advice to fight the pandemic.

Medical City Online, a UK based private sector Telehealth Software & Consultancy Company, teamed up with the government sector to launch Telemedicine-based initiatives such as Telemedicine 24/7 Helpline and subsequently Sehat Ghar Telemedicine Service. Such effort resulted in a significant number of tertiary hospitals across the country set up Telemedicine hubs to provide free of cost consultations across the country, serving over half a million beneficiaries. King Edward Medical University (KEMU) established remote consultation helpline accessible via "SKYPE". Every little help mattered as these initiatives formulated the backbone of the nation's response to the epidemic.

Ministry of National Health Services, Regulations and Coordination (MoNHSRC) launched a web portal called Yaaran-e-Watan focussed on attracting diaspora to help people of their country in providing free of cost consultations.

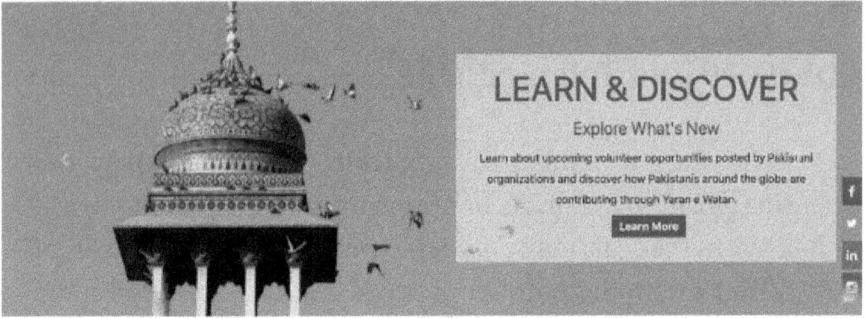

Sehat Kahani, a private sector Telehealth service provider, was taken on board to provide free of cost consultations to COVID-19 patients.

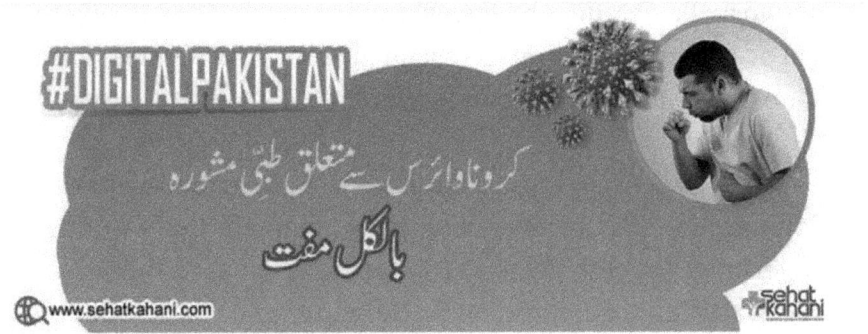

The biggest Mobile Health provider of the country Milvik Pakistan (JAZZ BIMA) was also taken on board to provide free of cost consultations pertaining to COVID-19. Their team of qualified doctors remained available 24/7 to provide Mobile Health services to citizens of Pakistan.

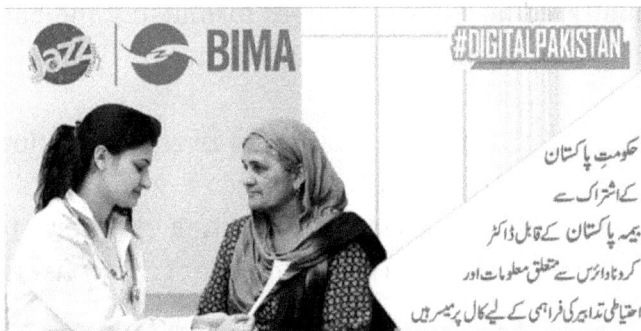

Our National helpline 1166 was manned with doctors to provide consultations to patients, WhatsApp Bot was launched to provide necessary symptomatic information to users and filter them for one-on-one consultations with the doctor.

Furthermore, Islamabad administration partnered with HealthPass Pakistan to equip Track, Trace and Quarantine (TTQ) teams in providing remote consultations to suspects identified during visits. The initiative was acclaimed and proven to be extremely useful in identifying patients for quarantine or sampling.

According to an estimate of MoNHSRC, more than 2 million Telemedicine and Mobile Health consultations were conducted in the last four months. The numbers speak for the uptake of technology and value proposition of initiatives.

Telemedicine is now an established reality and has been identified as one of the key areas for investment and focus. Programs are now designed around Telemedicine where the government is focussed on devising rules of business and support practitioners via legislation.

Mr Saflain Haider

Lead of the Health Informatics Wing – Ministry of National Health Services Regulation & Coordination

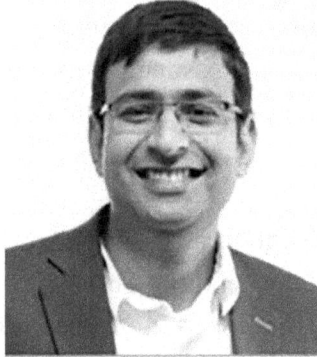

Saflain Haider holds a first degree from Middlesex University and completed his post-graduation from Kingston University. Haider carries an extensive experience of managerial roles at leading enterprises of Pakistan and the United Kingdom. Currently, he leads the Health Informatics Wing for Ministry of National Health Services Regulations and Coordination (MoNHSRC) as CIO for National Institute of Health (NIH). Haider represents MoNHSRC at National Command and Operation Centre (NCOC) and plays a pivotal role in defining tech strategy and providing support to federal and provincial governments. Haider has worked with gold partners of SAP, Tally Marks Consulting in Pakistan and MENA region as Director/Head of Project Delivery and rolled out SAP Audit Management and S4/HANA ERP centric solutions. Haider holds advisory positions for UNICEF and WHO as Deployment Specialist and Digital Health Expert, respectively.

Saflain Haider is also associated with Punjab - TEVTA as Digital Transformation Lead and is actively involved in the modernisation of traditional ways of teaching. He had been leading the E-Government Applications team at Punjab Information Technology Board (PITB) with his profound strategic planning, corporate branding, project management and business analytical skills. With more than fourteen years of professional experience, Saflain Haider has led the IT-centric healthcare reforms agenda for provincial and federal governments including deployment of Hospital Information Management System in DHQs and THQs, Automation of Drug Testing Labs, Telemedicine initiatives, EMR for Hepatitis and TB, Smartphone-based tracking for vaccinators (eVaccs), Online Bidding Platform for Local Purchase of Medicine and flagship projects of Dengue Surveillance and Integrated Disease Surveillance and Response (IDSR).

Saflain Haider led the first-ever rollout of HouseCall Doctors and designed the entire EMR and Billing flow for the client based out of Texas. He has been honoured by the Prime Minister of Pakistan and Chief Minister of Punjab, Minister for Health/Secretary Health and Chairman PITB for "Best Performance Award" against various initiatives on multiple occasions and served as a domain expert speaker for Management and Professional Development Department (MPDD) for public servants on healthcare IT.

Saflain Haider is a profound speaker with a bag full of successful talks and moderation experiences in various national and international conferences. Represented technological landscape of Government of Punjab and Government of Pakistan at various national and international forums and works actively with international partners to introduce sustainable innovation for the betterment of citizens.

Chapter Fourteen

COVID-19 and Social Determinants of Health

Economic and Social Conditions Influencing Healthcare

Author: Mr Jonathan M Fuchs, FACHE
Co. Author: Dr Suhail Chughtai

Introduction to the topic

The worldwide impact of the COVID-19 pandemic has exacerbated discrepancies in public health awareness, program activity and effectiveness. In particular, it highlighted the necessity to integrate Social Determinants of Health (SDOH) into the larger context of health care service and delivery, population health and policy.

Economic Conditions for an Optimum Healthcare

SDOH addresses the economic and social conditions that influence health statuses, such as physical environment, education, socioeconomic factors, social support, and access to healthcare services (1). Further, SDOH provides for an outsized effect on individual healthcare outcomes (2).

Social Requirements for Managing Healthcare

The Advisory Board, in particular, notes COVID-19's impact on SDOH worsens public health via food insecurity, housing instability, social isolation, and prejudice and discrimination (3). Adding to this are resource concerns of supply chain disruption of basic commodities, reduced access to primary care and delay of emergent care, and the general services disruption of often non-reimbursed or voluntary components of SDOH such as transportation, meals on wheels, and home healthcare. Each activity contributes to the toxic environment that COVID-19 intensifies.

Enhanced Role of Public Health Authorities

1. Public health authorities have long accepted the underlying environmental components of SDOH, which are integral to improving public health.
2. There is now recognition from healthcare systems, payors and governments that past inaction to address these discrepancies was unjustified.
3. Significant effort to recognise the need to support and fund SDOH activities must be placed front and centre as the pandemic decimates communities and families. Significantly affected are the poor and disadvantaged.
4. One is tempted to critique the various governmental attempts to confront and control the pandemic. Each country has had to address its own unique political and social environment-some with noted success others less so.
5. There remains controversy of approach and the availability of transparent, valid and accepted scientific and clinical information.

6. Inconsistent response or direction to public and media concerns toward prevention, treatment and vaccination serves only to allow COVID-19 to flourish unabated. It is imperative for clinicians, public health policy and epidemiologic professionals to be consistent, vigorous, and vocal to counter the disinformation and distrust.

An Opportunity to Upscale SDOH Services

The COVID-19 pandemic presents an essential opportunity to improve on how SDOH services are distributed, paid for, and monitored to enhance patient engagement and compliance.

It will prove to be an effort well spent to decelerate the COVID-19 spread, optimise treatment options, and ultimately improve the health and wellbeing of the population.

Gradual Incorporation of Telehealth & Telemedicine with Healthcare Systems

1879: Providing medical advice over telephone to reduce unnecessary clinic visits was mentioned in an article in Lancet.

1925: The cover of Science and Invention magazine showed a doctor diagnosing a patient by radio, visualising a device for a video examination of a patient over distance.

1948: Radiological images were sent via Telephone line covering 24 miles distance across the state of Pennsylvania, USA.

1959: Neurological examinations were transmitted for an Interactive Telemedicine service by the University of Nebraska, USA.

1959: Fluoroscopy images were sent across co-axial cable for diagnostic consultations by a Canadian Radiologist.
1960s: Closed Circuit TV link between Psychiatric Institute and Norfolk State Hospital was established for psychiatric consultations. US Space program sends animals biometric data to earth via Telemetric link.

Voice Radio Channels to transmit ECG rhythms from Fire Rescue Units to Jackson Memorial Hospital.

1970s: STARPAHC sets up "Space Technology Applied to Rural Papago Health Centre" connecting mobile support units in rural Tohono O'odham reservation link patients with Physicians in Indian Health Service Hospital.

Kaiser Foundation International and Lockheed Missiles and Space Company create a remote monitoring system capable of providing healthcare delivery.

1980s: Radiologists begin to use Teleradiology systems to receive images for providing opinion and reports.

1990s: Internet bandwidth permits a gateway for transmission of patient healthcare information across with larger data packets flourishing the concept of Telemedicine further with value proposition becoming more evident than before.

2010 and onward: The global Telehealth market size is projected to reach USD 266.8 billion by 2026, exhibiting a CAGR of 23.4% during the forecast period.

Rising adoption of Telehealth services to combat the rapid spread of the COVID-19 infection will play a key role in boosting market growth, finds Fortune Business Insights™ in its report, titled "Telehealth Market Share and Industry Analysis".

Telehealth leverages the power information and communication technology to provide remote healthcare services to patients.
By the end of 2018, seven million Americans will use Telehealth technology. Just five years ago, that number stood at 350,000. Analysts expect 100 million Telemedicine visits this year in the U.S.

The consumers of the service are now pushing the use of Telemedicine as indicated by an American patient survey from the nationwide chain of CVS Minute Clinics which reported up to a 99% satisfaction score with their Telehealth visit.

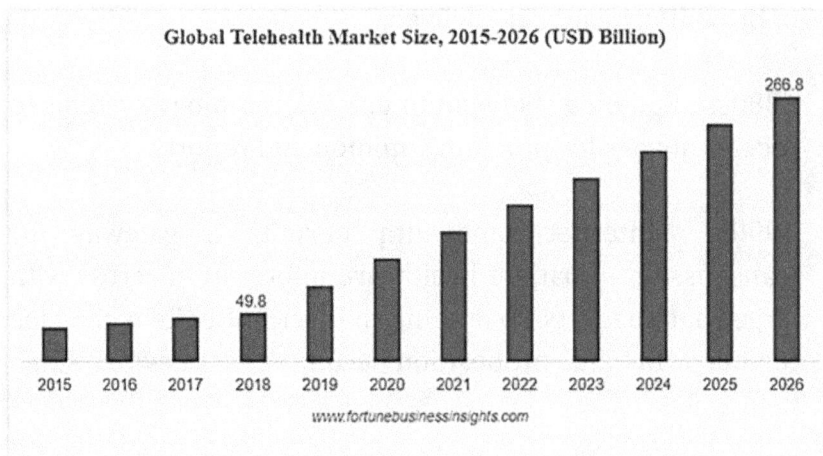

Global Telehealth Market Size, 2015-2026 (USD Billion)

266.8

49.8

2015 2016 2017 2018 2019 2020 2021 2022 2023 2024 2025 2026

www.fortunebusinessinsights.com

References

Heiman, H. J., and Artiga, S. (2015). Beyond health care: the role of social determinants in promoting health and health equity. Health 20, 1–10.

McFarlane, C; Finch, M; Gray, T; Fuchs, J; Hersh, W; Clouse, J. Incentivizing Change Within Social Determinants of Health Using Blockchain Technology. Front. Blockchain, 25 September 2020 | https://doi. org/10.3389/fbloc.2020.00040.

Sullivan, D; Connelly, E. Why COVID-19 could make social determinants of health even worse. Advisory.com/, daily-briefing/2020/03/25-sociaaldeterminants.

Abrams, E. and Szefler, S, COVID and the impact of social determinants of health. The Lancet.com/respiratory Vol 8 July 2020 p659-661

https://www.who.int/emergencies/diseases/novel-coronavirus-2019

Mr Jonathan M Fuchs *FACHE*

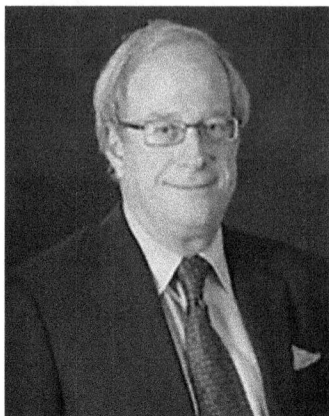

Mr Fuchs is the Chief Operating Officer of The Kidder Street Consulting Group, a US-based IT and HIT consultancy. He is a veteran health care executive with significant experience in managed care, health care management and operations.

His current consulting activity is focused on assisting health care start-up companies with developing reimbursement strategies, payment reform and the impact of data analytics/population health on value-based care.

Mr Fuchs is a Fellow in the American College of Healthcare Executives. He has a MA in college and university administration and a MS degree in health services administration. He serves on numerous advisory boards for health care start-up companies and currently serves on the Board of Directors of the Patientory Association.

Chapter Fifteen

How our Telemedicine Services Model can help other countries?

Suggestions with special reference to the National Health Service in the UK

Authors: Prof Angus Wallace & Dr Suhail Chughtai
Co-Authors: Ms Jumel Grace Ola, Dr Amir Michael &
Mr Graeme Allen

Telemedicine can make a difference to National Statistics
Amnesty Report on "Failure to Protect Healthcare
Professionals in the Pandemic"
Pakistan's response to COVID-19 pandemic as compared
with other countries

- Rallying official government and academic support
- The process of setting up a Telemedicine service
- Arranging a supply of doctors at the Telemedicine hub
- Training of the doctors
- Funding the project
- Team formation
- Spreading the word
- Audit and Quality Control

Introduction

The effect of the COVID-19 illness that became a pandemic from March 2020 has been to change the way health care needs to be delivered completely. For four months (March to June 2020) the provision of elective or planned health care in the UK was effectively suspended and, from the autumn of 2020 it had become clear that new and different ways of delivering health care are now required, and the protection of health care staff now has to be addressed far more seriously.

This chapter is being written when the second wave of COVID-19 disease has hit the UK and with the NHS having accumulated a huge backlog of unmet medical care needs including cancer patients, stroke and cardiac patients and, at the bottom of the pile, patients crippled by musculoskeletal diseases including osteoarthritis and other degenerative diseases that typically require joint replacement surgery.

The ongoing need for Telecare facilities during and after COVID-19 in the UK

There is now an ongoing challenge to address the backlog of NHS hospital patients that need to be seen, evaluated and either added to waiting lists if justified by their symptoms, or removed from waiting lists if their condition has changed. It has become clear from our Pakistan experience that using Telemedicine and Telecare might need to be further promoted, not only to manage this second wave but also to help address the NHS backlog significantly and to provide new ways of delivering a more efficient NHS service now more remote from the patient. Having experienced the first wave of COVID-19 and now (in November 2020) having moved into the second wave, there is an urgent need to ensure that Telemedicine is up and running efficiently in the UK with the skills and training of healthcare staff developed to use the technology appropriately. Face to face contact between the public and healthcare workers continues to be significantly risky, and the universal use of face masks is already creating communication problems. It can be argued that carrying out a Telemedicine consultation without face coverings is potentially a better method of communicating than a face-to-face consultation with both the healthcare staff and the patients wearing masks. In addition, the expense of providing Personal Protective Equipment (PPE) is avoided by a Telemedicine consultation with cost savings as a result. Once COVID-19 is under control the catch-up challenge of the backlog of NHS work will be immense, and this can also be addressed, even in the midst of a second wave, using both first referral and follow-up Telemedicine clinics.

Rallying official government and academic support

We recommend that government officials who support the use of Telemedicine and like the ideas presented in the earlier chapters of this book should be approached and invited to employ a "bottom-up" approach (as described in Chapter 10). These individuals would be the champions of Telemedicine. They would provide their support - both verbal and practical support as has occurred in Pakistan with the Governor of Punjab and indeed the Prime Minister, Imran Khan. These supporters would provide vital sustenance for a UK drive for this project.

In Pakistan, we found it was important to get the relevant key government officials supporting the daily medicine hotline because of several logistic hurdles including the Pakistan lockdown, social distancing policy and resistance from other parties who saw the development of Telemedicine as a threat. Although there can be problems reaching out to peripheral Telemedicine hubs, once some of the major hospitals and General Practitioner practices become committed, these will act as "lighthouses" demonstrating the practicality and commercial benefits of extending Telemedicine for the benefit of patients. One ideal way forward is to establish many Telemedicine hubs that will demonstrate to others how it can be done quickly and efficiently.

Academic support from medical schools and teaching hospitals is essential as there is currently a neglected need to train doctors and healthcare staff on the techniques required for an effective Telemedicine consultation. Hence, the support of key personnel in these areas is important. Many medical and legal pitfalls can occur with Telemedicine, and all these need to be addressed by staff training.

Once Telemedicine hubs are set up, users should be encouraged to talk about their experience, first booking their own appointment time on the internet, then waiting in the waiting room, seeing the specialist and then receiving their consultation note following the consultation on the same day (provided using a computer-based transcription) followed by the Consultant's letter with diagnosis and prognosis produced using Artificial Intelligence (AI) – all of which is now available.

Our experience in setting up the Doctors 24/7 Online Telemedicine hotline, highlighted the importance of trust between Vice-Chancellors of the various medical universities who collaborated. The Vice-Chancellor of one major University where the regional Telemedicine hub was created was Professor Dr Javaid Akram who made phone calls to several Vice-Chancellors from other universities of the province, and these worked wonders in creating multiple successful Telemedicine hubs after creating one in the central region of Punjab in the city of Lahore.

Having official support which we had in the form of the Governor of Punjab for Doctors 24/7 Online and the official academic support which the project had in the form of Professor Dr Javaid Akram, vice-Chancellor of the University of Health Sciences, Pakistan helped pave the way and provided the project with speed, often achieved with just one telephone call.

The changes in COVID-19 in the UK – November 2020 to 31 January 2021

COVID Vaccinations in the UK

The UK was the first country to approve COVID Vaccinations, first with the Pfizer/BioNTech vaccine on 2nd December 2020 and then with the Oxford/Astra Zenica vaccine on 30 December 2020 and the Moderna vaccine on 8th January 2021. As at 3st January 2021 vaccines from Janssen, Novavax and others are in the pipe-line but not yet approved.

The UK started its vaccination programme on 8th December 2020, focussing on the very elderly (over 80 years) first and the elderly (over 70 years) subsequently. By 29th January 2021 7.8 million people in the UK had been given their first COVID vaccination and of these approximately 0.5 million have also received their 2nd dose.

Known COVID Variants in the World

By January 2021 multiple variants of the virus that causes COVID-19 were found to be circulating globally.

The United Kingdom (UK) had identified a variant called B.1.1.7 with a large number of mutations in late 2020. This variant spreads more easily and quickly than other variants. In January 2021, experts in the UK reported that this variant may be associated with an increased risk of death compared to other variant viruses, but more studies are needed to confirm this finding. It has since been detected in many countries around the world. This variant was first detected in the US at the end of December 2020.

In South Africa, another variant called B.1.351 emerged independently of B.1.1.7. Originally detected in early October 2020, B.1.351 shares some mutations with B.1.1.7. Cases caused by this variant have been reported in the US at the end of January 2021.

In Brazil, a variant called P.1 emerged that was first identified in travellers from Brazil, who were tested during routine screening at an airport in Japan, in early January. This variant contains a set of additional mutations that may affect its ability to be recognized by antibodies. This variant was first detected in the US at the end of January 2021.

These variants seem to spread more easily and quickly than other variants, which may lead to more cases of COVID-19. An increase in the number of cases will put more strain on health care resources, lead to more hospitalizations, and potentially more deaths.

So far, studies suggest that antibodies generated through vaccination with currently authorized vaccines recognize these variants. This is being closely investigated and more studies are underway.

Rigorous and increased compliance with public health mitigation strategies, such as vaccination, physical distancing, use of masks, hand hygiene, and isolation and quarantine, is essential to limit the spread of the virus that causes COVID-19 and protect public health.

A total of 11,094 likely hospital-acquired covid-19 cases have been reported in the first 24 days of January, the latest data available. This is already higher than any other month in the second and third waves of covid.

The implications for UK Telemedicine - November 2020 to 31 January 2021

Obviously, the fast roll-out of the vaccination programme has been heralded as a true saviour in the UK and the general public are getting excited about the possibility of life returning to normal with no face coverings and social distancing. Unfortunately, the reality is that COVID is here to stay for many years and the vaccinations are not 100% effective with efficacy between 50% and 95% being estimated. That means that people are still going to get infected, but in smaller numbers, and hospitals are still going to admit patients with COVID disease for treatment but hopefully they will be less ill than we have seen to date.

In addition we do have a problem with hospital acquired COVID infection and at 29th January 2021 it was known that 450 patients per day caught COVID in hospitals during January.

This means that a long-term plan to reduce contact and prevent cross-infection is still required because there will still be infected people in the community and there is concern that the new variants of COVID listed above (and others in the future) may become resistant to the vaccinated patients.

We believe that the recommendations for increasing the use of Telemedicine referred to in Chapter 14 are even more required in the future to reduce the number of people attending hospital and to reduce the possibility of cross-infecting patients who are visiting or admitted to hospital with COVID.

We would therefore recommend the following:-

A strategy should be developed for triaging patients at home via Telemedicine who might have COVID before considering transferring them to hospital. This might be done by using a combination of assessment parameters such as those developed by Prof Tim Spector's Covid Symptom Study app [3] and the use of a remote pulse oximeter in the patient's home.

A strategy to reduce General Practitioner and hospital out-patient visits by using Telemedicine consultations as an alternative but with properly designed Medical Telemedicine platforms – not just video-meeting room consultation which fail to provide appropriate patient documentation and document transfer facilities.

Journey of Telemedicine from being a Product to a Service and stepping into becoming a Telehealth Culture.

Success of www.Doctors247.online as a successful Telemedicine remote healthcare delivery model, the Health Department of Punjab, the largest province with 110 million population formally approached Dr Suhail Chughtai to design a Telehealth Service Structure connecting Basic Health Unit in small towns and villages to the Specialist Doctors of District Headquarter Hospitals. The idea was to not only provide specialist care at the Basic Health Unit making life of the patient easy but also to off-load burden on District Hospitals OPD practice.

Dr Suhail Chughtai, designed a Telemedicine Service website, www.SehatGhar.online which was launched as a pilot in last quarter of 2020. Training of para-medical staff at the Basic Health Units and care-givers (Specialists) at the District Headquarter hospitals were trained in batches, both locally and by Dr Suhail Chughtai over e-class room. Till end of January, over 3000 patients have been treated by the Specialists through this website which has been deployed in Lahore Division of Punjab.

Amnesty Report on "Failure to Protect Healthcare Professionals in the Pandemic"

The Amnesty report on the UK Medical staff deaths during the first wave of the COVID-19 pandemic was published on 13th July 2020 - see

https://www.amnesty.org.uk/press-releases/uk-among-highest-COVID-19-health-worker-deaths-world

The summary of that report states –

UK among highest COVID-19 health worker deaths in the world

More than 540 health and social worker deaths in England and Wales, from 3,000 global fatalities

Health workers in Pakistan, Mexico and the Philippines attacked - others detained or dismissed for speaking out

It is tragic that we've seen so many of our dedicated healthcare workers in England and Wales die from COVID-19' - Kate Allen

The UK has recorded among the highest number of COVID-19 health worker deaths in the world, according to a new report by Amnesty International.

The 61-page report - Exposed, Silenced, Attacked: Failures to protect health and essential workers during the pandemic - shows that, with at least 540 health and social workers having died from COVID-19 in England and Wales alone, the UK is second only to Russia, which has recorded 545 health worker deaths.

Amnesty has collated and analysed a wide range of available data showing that more than 3,000 health workers have died after contracting COVID-19 in 79 countries. However, the figure is likely to be a significant underestimate due to under-reporting. According to Amnesty's monitoring, the countries with the highest numbers of health worker deaths thus far, are Russia (545), UK (England and Wales: 540, including 262 social care workers), USA (507), Brazil (351), Mexico (248), Italy (188), Egypt (111), Iran (91), Ecuador (82) and Spain (63)."

It is possible that more widespread use of Telemedicine in the UK, similar to the way it was used in Pakistan, might have reduced these 540 health and social worker deaths in England and Wales. It is important that this is considered and explored in the future.

The Process of setting up a Telemedicine Service

Setting up Telemedicine services involves a number of steps which are listed below:

Medical or Healthcare Professionals for providing Teleconsultation

In Pakistan, the most suitable healthcare staff were considered to be the young and middle-aged medical professionals, because of the recognised risk to elderly staff from COVID-19.

However, in the UK, the training of middle-aged and elderly staff for Teleconsultations has become more critical and should be considered a priority. It is also important to appreciate that those who contract COVID-19 often have minor symptoms, are not terribly unwell, and can still work on a virtual platform from their own home. The flexibility of Teleconsultations means that they can be carried out anytime during the day. For many patients, this is a real bonus because they can have their consultation outside of their regular working hours, and medical staff can be rostered appropriately to provide the most accommodating time for their patients.

For our Pakistan based COVID-19 acute service, we found young healthcare staff were more appropriate because they worked from designated hubs and had to travel using public transport to get there, thus being exposed to the risk of contracting COVID-19 during the hours of operation of the hubs and moving to and from the hub for an older colleague or more vulnerable healthcare provider. Working late nights, moving to and forth at odd hours of the day was also better tolerated by younger healthcare professionals as well. In the case of the Doctors 24/7 Telemedicine helpline, postgraduate medical trainees and young doctors doing their internship were invited to participate which they responded to very enthusiastically. Their contribution was recognised by providing appropriate Certificates and CPD points that were offered to support their ongoing studies or internship.

Telemedicine Software (usually cloud-based, therefore nothing to install)

We recommend Telemedicine software which is simple to understand and has a short learning curve. It should simulate the real doctor to patient encounter and should have the ability to incorporate PDF guidelines and PDF forms that inform the healthcare staff via the Telemedicine platform during the consultation. This facility, to provide guidelines and audit forms immediately will speed up the adoption of the Telemedicine platform by the doctors as a pre-set design of questions, will be guiding the medical professional through the Teleconsultation.

An Internet-connected PC

The PC's used in Pakistan for delivering the Telemedicine service was not "top of the range" but were considered "middle of the range" in relation to their specifications but had a dedicated internet connection with at least 1.0 MB upload and download speeds. This is well below the UK standards.

In Pakistan, the Internet connection was ideally through the Ethernet cable as Wi-Fi connexions could fluctuate and cause connection disruption between doctor and patient during a live Teleconsultation – this can also be a problem in the UK. The specification of the laptop computer should be at least two MB of ram with at least 1.8 gigahertz clock speed which is easily achievable through an i3 Intel or equivalent processor. The hard disc size may be moderate as minimal storage is required on the computer system itself, although it is advisable to have a minimum 20-inch size of monitor screen for providing the Telemedicine service. In NHS hospitals, careful consideration should be given to connectivity.

We do not recommend using the hospital-linked platforms because a combination of the delays in encryption and slow transmission speeds mean delays and interruptions to consultations can occur, and these can be very frustrating. The Telemedicine platform should include its own encryption (that should be NHS approved) but preferably not part of the NHS platform.

A suitable venue for the Medical Professionals (or working from home)

When creating a Telemedicine hub, a suitable room needs to be identified with suitably spaced computer stations, controlled temperature and appropriate air-conditioning to make the medical professionals feel comfortable while delivering their Telemedicine service. There should be suitable light on the face of the medical professional offering the service, and at the same time, the distance between two terminals should be enough to prevent crosstalk or overhearing for the sake of patient privacy.

Providing headphones and microphones is an option although patients have commented that "I'm not used to seeing a doctor with headphones on" and patients would be more comfortable speaking to a doctor as they would typically see them in clinics without headphones. Headphones are advised where the distance between the two terminals is not enough or when the microphones given to the doctors are not noise cancelling.

Tailoring an NHS venue needs to take into account the current Coronavirus guidance. The idea is to create well ventilated and suitably lighted large cubicles with sound insulation that would allow the attending doctor to carry out their consultation with the patient without having to apply a face covering or face mask. If hospital regulations require all medical staff to use masks, it is important to have this rule modified for those providing Telemedicine consultations if possible. The cubicle must be large enough to accommodate three screens, as shown in Figure 15.1 below.

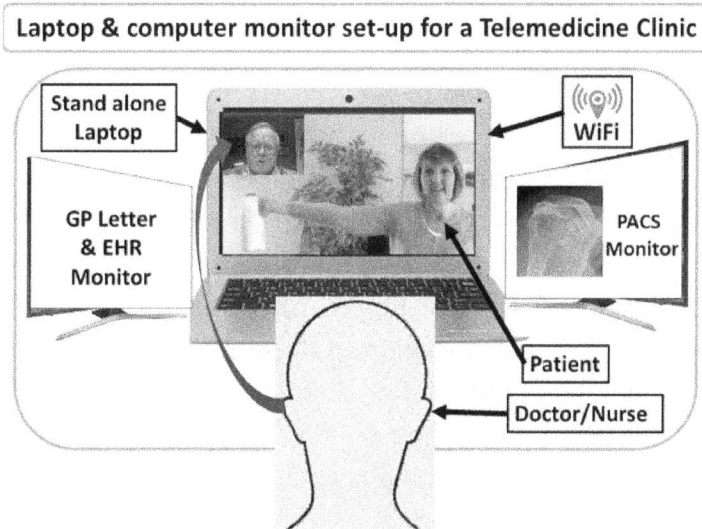

Laptop & computer monitor set-up for a Telemedicine Clinic

Stand alone Laptop

WiFi

GP Letter & EHR Monitor

PACS Monitor

Patient

Doctor/Nurse

Travelling for the doctors and health care staff to and from the Telemedicine hub should be supported by the official transport arrangements. It is possible that if the doctors have suitable facilities at home (laptop computer + broadband connections + a suitable room without interruptions from family members or pets), they can become part of the virtual Telemedicine hub from their home thus not requiring to travel.

Arranging a supply of doctors at the Telemedicine hub

This can be arranged through an automatic rota system, with half days allocated for Telemedicine consultations. It is not a good idea to mix real face-to-face consultations with Telemedicine consultations in a clinic area because of the setting up of the equipment and the risk of breach of privacy if you have patients present in the room at any stage of a Telemedicine consultation.

Training the doctors and healthcare professionals to run Telemedicine

To deliver an efficient service, the staff requires to be trained to use the Telemedicine software. Such training in Pakistan was provided to the doctors through intermittent webinars on their terminals along with in-person local coordinators at each Telemedicine hub for on the spot troubleshooting. This training not only minimised the learning curve but also kept the doctors motivated during their period of service. In the UK intermittent webinars should be instituted, and tutorials should focus on how to use the Telemedicine platform efficiently and how to carry out a remote consultation so that the patient is provided with the best consultation possible.

These tutorials will need to focus on how medical staff should position themselves, how they adjust their lighting and background, how to behave, how to act with good and bad news and how to involve other people, i.e., the patient's family member or a friend in the consultation. The hospital staff will also need guidance on the best documentation for their consultation, how the computer-based transcription of the consultation and how the consultation letter produced with AI (Artificial Intelligence) has been designed. This should create a letter that is automatically populated with diagnosis, prognosis and follow-up arrangements after the consultation has been completed.

Innovation in the venue for patients to attend Virtual Consultations

We now have an opportunity to be innovative in a relatively inexpensive way. The NHS should consider setting up Virtual Consultation Rooms in locations that are suitable for the general public in a similar way to the changes being made by the Post Office and Banks. Why should we not set up Consultation cubicles with smart measuring devices for body weight, temperature, pulse, ECG, heart auscultation, and imaging tools within stores or supermarkets in the UK and linked virtually to NHS hospitals. These would give the public easier and more convenient access to healthcare in a much more efficient and friendly way. While the COVID-19 pandemic is still active, it would also reduce the need for PPE for hospital staff, although the Consultation Room Nurse or attendant would still require it.

Barriers to Effective Implementation of Telehealth Services within the NHS

Our co-author, Ms Jumel Grace Ola, is a USA Hospital Administrator from Chicago, who has just completed her master's degree in business administration at Durham University, UK, on "Facilitators and Barriers to Virtual Health Implementation in the UK".

Her research showed that there are many barriers to effective implementation of virtual health care services in the UK, including digital exclusion, lack of IT support, and connectivity issues in remote areas.

Various obstacles are present that prevent the optimal implementation of virtual health services. One critical barrier is the security risk regarding personal data that is exchanged between the patient and clinicians (Torous et al., 2020). The legal liability of data leakage can create financial problems. A data breach is a serious concern that could cost a large health care organisation millions of pounds in fines, not to mention, the loss of reputation. Patients trust healthcare organisations to protect their confidential information, including medical history and other private information. Online attacks can take many forms. One is a ransomware attack where hackers prevent access to data unless a ransom is paid (Young & Yung, 2017). Other barriers that have been identified by researchers include the preference of healthcare consultants for face-to-face interaction, resistance to a change in management practices, and administration issues (Bradford et al., 2016).

Financial constraints, including long and short-term funding, are also a key barrier in the implementation of virtual health services (Fisk et al., 2020). Poor internet connections in remote areas also serve as an obstacle to the implementation of virtual health care services (Fisk et al., 2020).

Digital exclusion has been quite a challenge. About 5 million households are offline and do not have internet in the UK, and nearly 75% of UK residents without an internet connection are over 60 years old (Wyatt, 2019). Statistics show that individuals are three times more likely to be digitally excluded if they are from a lower socioeconomic, low literacy background or if they have a disability (accuRx, 2020). Digital exclusion is also impacted by language, income, literacy, ethnicity, and culture (Ray, Stevens, & Thirunavukarasu, 2020). There is a close correlation between the digital exclusion of health care services and lower socioeconomic status (NHS, 2019).

Around 50 % of individuals in the UK without a net connection have income that is below the poverty line, while 64 % live in rural areas (Shropshire Council, 2016). Patients suffering from vision or hearing impairments may also have difficulties in accessing health care services (Hjelm, 2005). It is crucial to identify this small population because if we are not cautious, this could be the small percentage that could drive up healthcare costs due to not having the means to use virtual health care services for their preventative care.

Bureaucratic difficulties act as an obstacle to the implementation of virtual health care services (Hjelm, 2005). Privacy and security are essential aspects of building trust and confidence in virtual health care systems (Nikus et al., 2009). But no standard practices or regulatory mechanisms are present regarding the coverage of liability for the patients in the case of virtual health services (Rafiq & Merrell, 2005).

On 20th March 2020, Sir Simon Stevens, Chief Executive Officer, NHS England issued an instruction that the Control of Patient Information (COPI) Regulations (2002) were to be suspended until 30th September 2020 (NHS 2020a) to permit the exchange of information more freely within health trusts to facilitate NHS staff digital communication during the COVID-19 pandemic period and thus maximise their staffing resources and quality of care delivered to their constituencies. This period has been further extended in August 2020 to 31st March 2021 (NHS 2020b), and this extension does facilitate the ongoing provision of Telemedicine services in the UK at present. Without future well-thought-out COPI regulations, interoperability will remain a barrier to Telehealth services in the UK.

Lackofbroadbandaccessisabarriertotheimplementation of virtual healthcare services in remote areas in the UK. Many rural areas in the UK have inadequate broadband services. A 2013 report from Ofcom – the communication regulatory authority in the UK – found that nearly 5 % of the population are without broadband access of at least 2 Mbps of which majority were from rural areas (Townsend, Sathiaseelan, Fairhurst, & Wallace, 2013).

Funding the project

This major obstacle was resolved in Pakistan by deploying the medical professionals, which were offered continuous medical education as their incentive. In the UK, the doctors and healthcare staff would be working on a formally employed basis. If they are working from home, a full document of their hours of work must be carried out and approved by their employer.

Team Formation

The organisation of the Telemedicine Team is really important. In Pakistan the project team was divided into the following layers:

- The regional Telemedicine hub coordinator
- The regional logistic coordinator
- The regional Telemedicine trainer
- The regional Duty roster coordinator

Besides the original team, there was a central project coordinator team which consisted of the following:

- The project lead coordinator
- The project quality control in charge
- The lead Telemedicine Instructor

- The central liaison officer
- The project spokesperson for press and media
- The project marketing advisor

For doctors 24/7 Telemedicine helpline, the project secretariat was based at the University of Health Sciences with one operating room at the governor of Punjab's office. For the UK a clear structure for the team will need to be developed to cover the creation of Telemedicine rotas, the method of allocating time slots for patients to book themselves, the coordination of the patient's EHR (Electronic Health Record), the GP referral letter and any investigations such as x-rays and scans that may be required. We recommend that the consulting doctor works from at least two screens – one with the patient's EHR and access to test results, a second screen for the PACS (Picture Archiving Communication System) screen for x-rays and scans and the Telemedicine platform screen.

Spreading the word

The project awareness in the common public is the key to success. Several means can be used involving print and press along with social media. Involvement of key public figures, including politicians, film industry, sports and other national heroes serves as a fast means to get the message across. In case of the Pakistan "doctors 24/7" platform, the help of media stars and famous politicians were taken to get the word out in the form of short messages on social media and advertisements on the TV channel.

Audit and Quality Control

Reports should be set up early to evaluate the usage of the system. In Pakistan, we arranged a weekly audit of the "doctors 24/7 Telemedicine helpline" which showed the number of patients advised through the helpline and also gave a statistical analysis of the disease burden which helped to identify hotspots of the infection and thus identified the epidemic spread based on symptoms alone. This guided the government and allowed them to take appropriate measures. The figures also indicated a progressive decrease in certain zones as compared to rising disease burden in others which indicated the vulnerable geographical spots in the country. Hopefully, in the UK, we will be running the Telemedicine platforms predominantly for non-coronavirus patients. So the focus will be on the management of elective cases. Still, these would be audited based on medical or surgical speciality, age of the patient, diagnosis and action, i.e. placed on a waiting list or referred for investigation or specific treatment.

References

accuRX, 2020. accuRx Webinar: Accessible Design and Digital Inclusion in Health care. [Youtube Video]. https://www.youtube.com/watch?v=ReiGZYp0QyM&feature=emb_err_woyt

Bradford, N., Caffery, L., & Smith, A. (2016). Telehealth services in rural and remote Australia: A systematic review of models of care and factors influencing success and sustainability. Rural and Remote Health, 16, 3808. https://doi.org/10.22605/RRH3808

Fisk, M., Livingstone, A., & Winona, S. (2020). Telehealth in the Context of COVID-19: Changing Perspectives in Australia, the United Kingdom, and the United States. Journal of Medical Internet Research 22(2), e19264. https://doi.org/10.2196/19264

Hjelm, N.M. (2005). Benefits and drawbacks of Telemedicine. Journal of Telemedicine & Telecare. 11(2), 60-70. https://doi.org/10.1258/1357633053499886

NHS (2019). Digital inclusion matters to health and social care organisations https://digital.nhs.uk/about-nhs-digital/our-work/digital-inclusion/digital-inclusion-in-health-and-social-care

NHS (2020a) COVID-19 – Notice under Regulation 3(4) of the Health Service Control of Patient Information Regulations 2002 https://www.england.nhs.uk/publication/COVID-19-notice-under-regulation-34-of-the-health-service-control-of-patient-information-regulations-2002/

NHS (2020b) COVID-19 – Control of patient information (COPI) notice https://digital.nhs.uk/coronavirus/coronavirus-COVID-19-response-information-governance-hub/control-of-patient-information-copi-notice

Nikus, K., Lähteenmäki, J., Lehto, P., & Eskola, M. (2009). The role of continuous monitoring in a 24/7 telecardiology consultation service--a feasibility study. Journal of Electrocardiology, 42(6), 473-480. https://doi.org/10.1016/j.jelectrocard.2009.07.005

Rafiq, A., &Merrell, R.C. (2005). Telemedicine for access to quality care on medical practice and continuing medical education in a global arena. Journal of Continuing Education in the Health Professions, 25(1), 34-42. https://doi.org/10.1002/chp.7

Ray, A., Stevens, A., & Thirunavukarasu, A. (2020). Offline and left behind: how digital exclusion has impacted health during the COVID-19 pandemic. https://blogs.bmj.com/bmj/2020/07/03/offline-and-left-behind-how-digital-exclusion-has-impacted-health-during-the-COVID-19-pandemic/

Torous, J., Jän, M. K., Rauseo-Ricupero, N., & Firth, J. (2020). Digital mental health and COVID-19: using technology today to accelerate the curve on access and quality tomorrow. JMIR Mental Health 7(3): e18848

Townsend, L., Sathiaseelan, A., Fairhurst, G. & Wallace, C. (2013). Enhanced broadband access as a solution to the social and economic problems of the rural digital divide. Local Economy: The Journal of the Local Economy Policy Unit, 28(6), 580-595. https://doi.org/10.1177/0269094213496974

Wyatt, T. (2019). More than five million British people have never used the internet, official figures reveal. Independent. https://www.independent.co.uk/news/uk/home-news/internet-use-uk-national-how-many-people-a8806806.html

Young, A. L., & Yung, M. (2017). Privacy and security cryptovirology: The birth, neglect, and explosion of ransomware: recent attacks exploiting a known vulnerability continue a downward spiral of ransomware-related incidents. Communications of the ACM, 60(7), 24-26. https://doi.org/10.1145/3097347

Miss Jumel Grace Ola

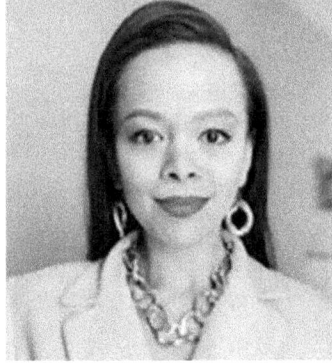

Jumel Grace Ola, MBA, MPH is a public health administrator who has had 15 years of experience in healthcare working in various settings clinical, research, patient education and health policymaking. Jumel is also the Telehealth Business Administrator for Medical City Online, UK.

She received her bachelor's degree in biology from San Francisco State University. She obtained her master's degree in public health at The Chicago School of Professional Psychology and completed her master's degree in business administration at Durham University Business School, UK where she wrote a dissertation on "The Facilitators and Barriers to Virtual Health Implementation in the UK".

Dr Amir Michael

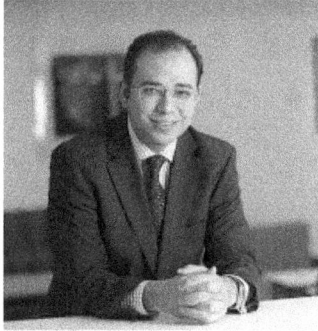

Associate Professor (Teaching) in Accounting/Programme Director
Full-time MBA in the Business School
Telephone: +44 (0) 191 33 40222

Contact Dr Amir Michael (email at a.e.iskander@durham.ac.uk)
www.dur.ac.uk/research/directory/staff/?mode=staff&id=5161

Dr Amir Michael is an Associate Professor (Teaching) in Accounting at Durham University Business School, Durham University, UK and director of the Durham MBA (FT) Programmed. Dr Michael is the director of the Durham Rutgers Accounting Analytics Network (DRAAN). Amir's research and teaching interests have been fostered by several years of undergraduate and postgraduate teaching and mentoring. His research interest comprise a variety of areas in the Accounting and Auditing profession including, Using Big Data Analytics and Artificial Intelligence in Auditing and Forensic Investigations, Accounting information Systems, Voluntary Reporting, Corporate Governance and Accounting Education. He serves on the editorial board of the Journal of Emerging Technology in Accounting.

Mr Graeme Allen

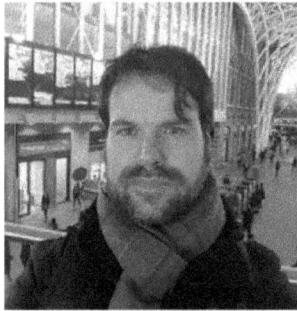

Senior Project Manager at North of England Commissioning Support
Contact Graeme Allen at graeme.allen2@nhs.net

Graeme is a Senior Project Manager working within technology, transformation and innovation with the National Health Service (NHS). He has over 15 years experience in IT-related projects across the public and private sectors working on delivering information systems, office moves, fibre broadband installations and web-based projects based on Business Analysis programmes and system integration.

He currently works for a CSU with the NHS as Senior Project Manager where his main role is to work on National Projects which have been commissioned from NHSE. This involves good communications as work with the National team to establish deliveries, acceptance criteria and governance so I have channels established to feedback and link into stakeholders. He is responsible for leading, planning and delivering numerous strategic projects, including the national programme for IT.

For the service he investigates new opportunities and liaises with a wide diversity of internal and external stakeholders to ensure that this service is delivered effectively and plays a key lead role in forging partnerships with and influencing peers.

He is an established relations with National technology groups which he attends and has presented at a number of National meetings and events. He has worked with National technology initiatives regarding technical discussions around standards such as SNOMED, FHIR and IHE to suggest options on a code that could be used by all within healthcare and future proof digital services.

He has developed effective client relationship with internal and external stakeholders and uses market knowledge to build up a comprehensive understanding of the project, understand best practice and alternative methods so that an effective plan can be drafted which supports efficiency.

He has NHS I have worked for other organisations:

- NHS Business Service Authority (NHSBSA) Provided hands-on support and leadership for the development and implementation of projects, working closely with the relevant areas of the business to work towards delivering the Pacific goals of saving one billion pounds across the NHS.

- NHSE as a Project Manager with the Interoperability team, managed the National project for digital cancer. A large part of this work involved linking together a number of on-going initiatives to prevent duplication of effort. The end result included a recommendation report on a number of areas that went to the National Cancer Director.

He has worked in the NHS at local and national level and have therefore witnessed the positive and negative aspects of the NHS. At the heart of it all though, witnessed the drive to make a change and keep the NHS running effectively as possible. His career goal would be to continue this drive using innovation and technology across the full landscape of the NHS which will include mental health to volunteer organisations joining up and sharing best practice and working together.

Specialties: Information technology, project management, digital, change management, networking, user journeys, Prince2, Business analysis, Primavera, Forex day trading.

Chapter Sixteen

Getting together and working in Harmony for the Project

Tribute to the Operations Team of the Telemedicine Helpline

Author: *Dr Suhail Chughtai*

The Doctors 24/7 Online Telemedicine Project Team

TEAM - GOVERNOR HOUSE PUNJAB

• Chaudhary Mohammad Sarwar	Project Lead and Patron in Chief
• Ms Rabia Zia	Chief Coordinator Planning Meetings
• Chaudhary Ansar Farooq	Coordinator Logistics & Maintenance

TEAM - UNIVERSITY OF HEALTH SCIENCES

• Prof Dr Javed Akram	Primary Telemedicine Hub Incharge
• Dr Khurram Shahzad	Incharge Coordination & Deployment
• Dr Humayun Taimur Baig	Incharge Project Service Operations
• Prof Dr Nasir Shah	Incharge Doctor's Training Coordination

• Dr Saqib Mehmood	Coordinator, UHS based Logistics
• Dr Asad Zaheer	Coordinator, UHS based Logistics
• Mr Asif Mehmood	Incharge Web Portal Admin
• Mr Farhan Ahmed	Incharge Ground Logistics

TEAM – MEDICAL CITY ONLINE

• Dr Suhail Chughtai	Lead Software Designer & Instructor
• Deputy Software Instructors	Dr Sohaib Imtiaz, Dr Ahmed Ejaz, Dr Salman Shafi, Dr Syed Ali
• Mr Jamal Abdul Wahid	Process Coordinator
• Web Development – Quality Control	A team of 3 experienced professionals

Dr KHURRAM SHAHZAD (Incharge Project Coordination & Deployment)

- Emergency Medicine Physician Ireland (Locum)
- Visiting Consultant and Project Director (Volunteer) of Institute of Learning Emergency Medicine – ILEM, University Health Sciences, Pak
- CEO International Institute of Learning Medicine – IILM
- Convener (Volunteer), Department of Telemedicine and Health Informatics, University of Health Sciences, Lahore, Pakistan
- Focal Person and Consultant (Volunteer) National Patient Referral Program UHS

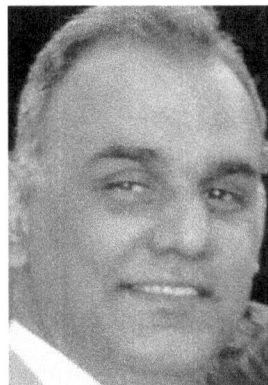

- Ex Advisor to Chairman Pakistan Red Crescent Society
- Ex Regional Director of College of Physicians and Surgeons Pakistan in Ireland
- Founder of Disaster Relief by Irish and Pakistanis D.R.I.P. Ireland.
- Founding Director and Faculty member (Volunteer) of National Ambulance College Pakistan IILM (Branches in EDHI, PRCS, RESCUE 1122) in Collaboration with NAS Dublin and UCD Ireland
- Lead Consultant for National Disaster Management vision 2030

Dr Shahzad took the key responsibility of Project Coordination, ensuring a seamless blend of individual units operating in sync. The job was not only concentration intensive but also required frequent travelling from Lahore to other cities at short notice to set up several secondary Telemedicine Hubs upon taking up several medical institutions of Punjab as service delivery partners in this project.

During the periods of lockdown, special arrangements were needed to travel between cities which at times was stressful, though his dedication and selfless drive helped achieve the objectives. Within two weeks of the launch, Dr Shahzad managed to set up over 21 Secondary Telemedicine Hubs through his tireless work in five medical universities and 16 Health and Allied Health facilities in the provinces of Punjab, Baluchistan and KPK.

He also ensured that the groups adhered to updated SOPs through timely information sharing across 21 WhatsApp groups requiring significant time. He developed FAQs about the operational steps for the doctors without incurring any cost to the University.

Dr Shahzad's experience of working within government rules and disaster management helped in officially creating departments within 24 hours, with all relevant Government permissions. He received full support from Prof Dr Javed Akram, the VC UHS and Governor Punjab, the Chancellor UHS. Dr Shahzad was instrumental in managing the following tasks:

- Designing SOPs, the Standard Operating Procedures
- Training program for the volunteering doctors
- Funding sources (operational costs)
- Utility of existing resources
- Organisation of HR

Dr HUMAYOUN TEMOOR BAIG (Incharge Project Operations at UHS)

- Forensic Odontologist, Medico legal Punjab
- Senior Lecturer at the University of Health Sciences, Pakistan
- Board Member of Association of the Forensic Odontology for Human Rights
- Secretary-General of Global Dental Health & Education Alliance.

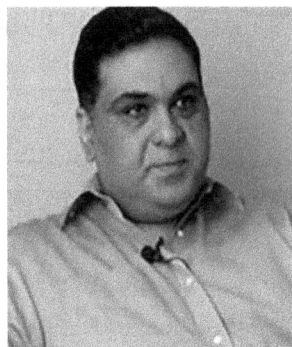

Dr Humayoun Baig, being the Operations Incharge, played a highly significant role in the project management. The quality of operations from the installation of stations, to doctor's 24/7 roster formation, their training sufficiency, adherence to the designed roster and then quality control of the service, all fell in his domain of role.

Dr Baig possessed that eye for detail required for supervising the execution of major operative steps in the process of conducting around the clock Telemedicine Helpline.

Prof Dr ABDUL NASIR SHAH (Incharge Doctor's Training Coordination)

* Head Department of Family Medicine & Primary Healthcare, University of Health Sciences, Pakistan
* Consultant Family Physician, Lahore, Pakistan

Prof Nasir Shah set up and coordinated the training sessions of over 350 doctors that went through the Software Training program. Dr Suhail Chughtai instructed live Telemedicine Workshops over *www.Videoroom.online,* a medical-grade training software of Medical City Online.

Auditorium and Training rooms of the University of Health Sciences were used for the purpose. Prof Dr Nasir Shah devoted significant effort to ensure a quality training medium available to the doctors.

Dr SAQIB MEHMOOD   Head of Education Dept, UHS
DR ASAD ZAHEER   Registrar UHS

Both senior Medical Professionals of the University of Health Sciences supported the project by giving back up admin support to any logistic issues faced. The admin work such as approvals, goods release etc., was facilitated at a fast pace to ensure that both the setting up and maintenance of the Telemedicine Helpline project remained smooth all the way.

Mr ASIF MEHMOOD   Incharge Web Portal Admin

Mr Mehmood, a devoted member of the time right from the inception of the project was trained by the Medical City Online's London office team to manage the backend of the website locally in terms of setting Doctor's Login and Icons. Also, Mr Mehmood was the Incharge of data compilation for audit and statistical analysis.

Mr FARHAN AHMED   Incharge Ground Operations Logistics

Mr Farhan Ahmed was deputed to manage operations facilitating the Telemedicine Service such as commuting arrangements of female doctors at night shift, food/snacks for the on-duty doctors, ensuring computers and internet facility worked flawlessly etc.

MS RABIA ZIA   Chief of the Staff, Governor House Punjab.

Ms Rabia Zia helped establish communication channels between the Governor Punjab and various teams interacting with the Governor's relevant team.

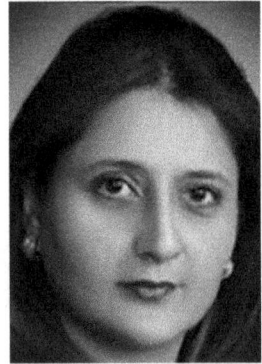

CHAUDHARY ANSAR FAROOQ Project Coordinator, Governor House Punjab, Pakistan

Chaudhary Farooq's role in coordinating for organising necessary logistics, especially for setting up the Telephone support to the Telemedicine project was regarded as highly valuable.

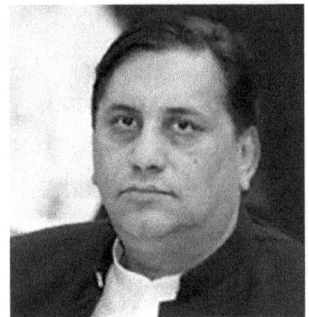

The Deputy Software Instructors

These young doctors were the first to be trained whom I did during one-on-one sessions, taking them through each screen. I was satisfied to see their eye for detail and was happy for them to be the local Software Instructors for day-to-day queries by the online doctors.

DR. SYED MUHAMMAD ALI
Senior Lecturer
Department of Pathology
Rawalpindi Medical University, Rawalpindi, Pakistan

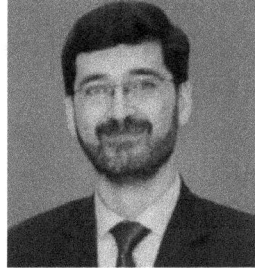

DR MUHAMMAD SOHAIB JAVED
BDS (de' Montmorency College of Dentistry), B.Sc. (Punjab University)
Resident Orthodontist (Royal Orth. Foundation Cairo)

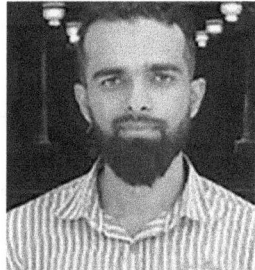

DR. AHMED EJAZ
House Officer
Arif Memorial Teaching Hospital
Lahore, Pakistan

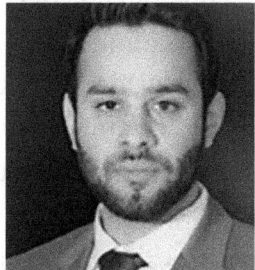

DR. SALMAN SHAFI KOUL
Assistant Professor of Critical Care Medicine
Shaheed Zulfiqar Ali Bhutto Medical University Islamabad, Pakistan

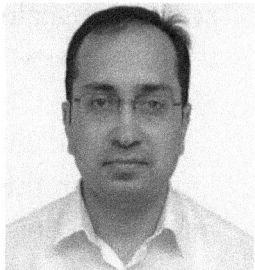

Comments of Support

Dr SYED TARIQ SHAHAB *MD, FACC, FACP*
Director Vascular and Interventional Cardiology
Clinical Associate Professor of Medicine (Cardiology)
George Washington University Hospital, Washington DC
Chairman, APPNA Fall Meeting 2018, Washington DC

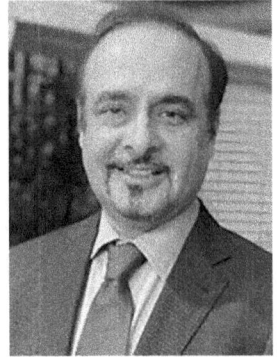

I congratulate both authors, Prof Angus Wallace and Dr Suhail Chughtai, who are UK based Orthopaedic Surgeons, for their book, "Telemedicine, a novel way to fight a pandemic". This healthcare success story from Pakistan, is a narrative of the journey of converting Telemedicine into an effective tool for connecting patients to doctors despite the restrictions of physical meeting between them.

Telemedicine was originally created to treat patients who were in remote places, far away from local health facilities or in areas with shortages of medical professionals. In 1922, Dr Hugo Gernsback featured the tele-dactyl in a science magazine. The first radiologic images were sent via telephone between two medical centers in Pennsylvania by 1948.

Dr Suhail Chughtai can easily be called a pioneer and key innovator in this field and his immense contribution needs no introduction. He was deservedly awarded "APPNA Award for Innovation in Telemedicine in 2018" at the annual event of this largest organization of overseas Pakistani Doctors

(APPNA), based in the USA.

Telemedicine has been through a striking evolution in the last decade and is becoming an increasingly important part of the global healthcare infrastructure. Recent policy changes during the COVID-19 pandemic have reduced barriers to tele-health access and have promoted the use of telehealth to deliver acute, chronic, primary and specialty care. However, Dr Suhail Chughtai had this vision even before the pandemic and has been instrumental in implementing tele medicine as a source of health care delivery not only in Pakistan, but Middle East and United Kingdom too.

I congratulate both Prof Angus Wallace and Dr Suhail Chughtai along with the Co-authors of this book which promises to bring a worthwhile contribution to the world of Telemedicine.

Prof Dr TANVIR KHALIQ
Vice Chancellor, Shaheed Zulfiqar Ali
Bhutto Medical University
Islamabad, Pakistan

Dr Fibhaa Syed
Assistant Prof in Medicine, Shaheed
Zulfiqar Ali Bhutto Medical University,
Islamabad, Pakistan

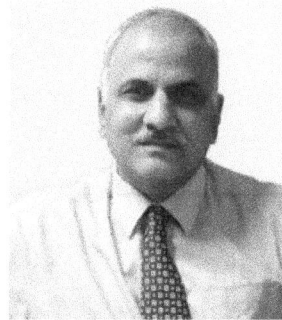

The initiative of telemedicine in Pakistan in the grave times of COVID19 pandemic served to unite the nation further in fighting the war against an enemy we knew nothing about. As doctors we felt we could alleviate our patients fears and anxiety at a time the world had shut its doors to patients.

We achieved the objective by using the Telemedicine Hotline set up by Dr Suhail Chughtai at www.Doctors247. online. We not only prevented many patients from unduly reaching out to the hospitals but were able to guide those who needed dire attention. The patients we interacted with through Doctors 24/7 Online website for Tele-consultations, felt extremely grateful and cared for.

Mr FEROZE DADA
Chartered Accountant, TV Interviewer
Founder Trustee Charity at The Inle Trust

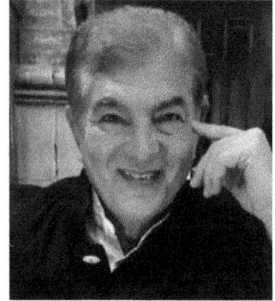

My dear Suhail, I remember very clearly the Sunday morning few years back when you call me at your home, making me the first person to witness the final design of your Telemedicine software. While you gave me a demo, I could sense the excitement you expressed with intention to make positive change for people's health.

No doubt the software was very inspiring but what impressed me at that time was not just the software. It was your courage to launch a product in the face of competition from the big companies and your determination to put this to use for a good cause. But as a wise man once said, "Be patient everything comes to you at the right moment"; and so it has.

Well done my friend and I wish you every success in helping humanity with your intellect & expertise in this difficult time of the Corona pandemic.

Best wishes

Prince MOHSIN ALI KHAN
Founding Chairman, World Peace &
Prosperity Foundation
London, UK

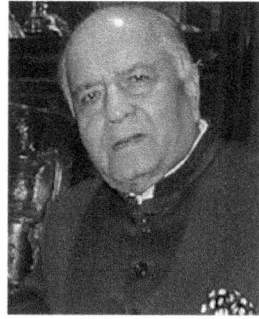

My dear Suhail, you always wanted to make people's lives better.

I am proud to know that your Telemedicine Technology is doing what you intended to use it for.

My organisation recognized your passion earlier in 2018 and duly awarded you our Annual Award at a ceremony in the House of Lords, Westminster, London for your services to help humanity in healthcare sector.

I wish you well in the pursuit of your journey and may you see further success.

Best wishes & love

Dr MUHAMMAD NADEEM KHAWAJA
Secretary General, DOCTORSCON
– Medical Organization of Family
Physicians, Pakistan

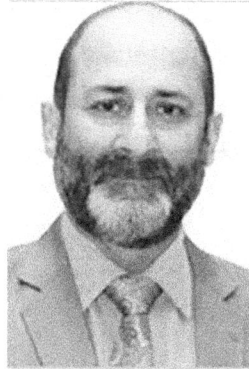

I was introduced to Telemedicine by Dr Suhail Chughtai 3 years ago. In Pakistan, the best thing was that Governor Sarwar and VC University of Health Sciences Lahore, Prof Javed Akram realized the importance of Telemedicine very early into the Corona epidemic.

Both the Governor and the VC facilitated Dr Suhail Chughtai resulting in an unprecedented number of patients getting treated through Telemedicine . Our organization DOCTORSCON , (premier Family medicine organization in Pakistan) , salutes this Pakistani Hero.

Dr MIAN TARIQ MEHMOOD
Chairman: Pakistan Academy of Family Physicians, Pakistan

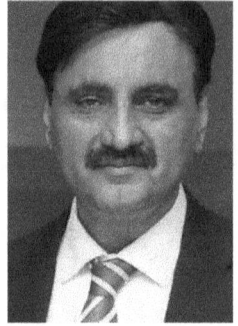

Delivery of healthcare through Telemedicine is an established channel however, COVID-19 epidemic in Pakistan took the understanding to a higher level. Dr Suhail Chughtai was deeply involved and led the project of Telemedicine Corona 24/7 Helpline by providing a Telemedicine Website and training to the doctors providing free medical advice through this service. He has also instructed Family Physicians of my organization through several short courses on Telemedicine.

I am convinced that role of Telemedicine is going to be gain further importance as doctors and patients get to use it more. At present, in Pakistan, several projects at national level have started incorporating Telemedicine as the alternative route of bringing healthcare to the patient's doorstep. I congratulate Dr Suhail Chughtai and Prof Angus Wallace on compiling their expertise in this book.

Lady Mayor, FRANCES STAINTON
Co. Chairperson, World Peace & Prosperity Foundation
London, UK

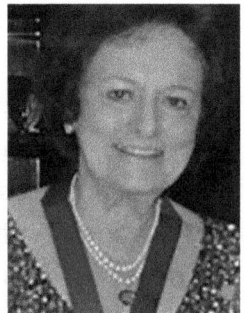

Dear Dr Chughtai, I am not surprised to see your Telemedicine technology delivering a purposeful service and making life of large number of people better. You always put passion in your projects which helps you get your results. I support your work and wish you further achievements. All the best.

Short Stories and Narratives of various people involved directly or indirectly with the Telemedicine Corona Helpline Project

4 Young Heroes, serving selflessly, exemplifying role of young doctors.

The 4 doctors sharing their experience of providing around the clock free medical advice on Doctors 24/7 Telemedicine Website as the Healthcare Volunteers of this project.

These young doctor's inspiring narrative shows the impact created by the project on young medical professionals.

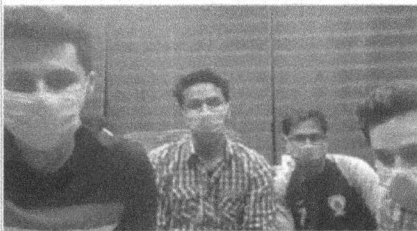

A young doctor helping across borders, beyond ethnic or religious divide.

Caring for others goes beyond borders and irrespective of ethnicity or religion. A young doctor shares her experience of examining a patient from India offering free medical advice during the Corona lockdown.

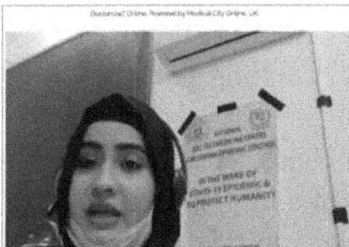

Chapter Seventeen

The changes in COVID-19 in the UK
November 2020 to 31 January 2021

Authors: Prof Angus Wallace & Dr Suhail Chughtai

COVID Vaccinations in the UK

The UK was the first country to approve COVID Vaccinations, first with the Pfizer/BioNTech vaccine on 2nd December 2020 and then with the Oxford/ Astra Zenica vaccine on 30 December 2020 and the Moderna vaccine on 8th January 2021. As at 31st January 2021, vaccines from Janssen, Novavax and others are in the pipeline but not yet approved.

The UK started its vaccination programme on 8th December 2020, focussing on the very elderly (over 80 years) first and the elderly (over 70 years) subsequently. By 29th January 2021 7.8 million people in the UK had been given their first COVID vaccination and of these approximately 0.5 million have also received their 2nd dose.

Known COVID Variants in the World

By January 2021 multiple variants of the virus that causes COVID-19 were found to be circulating globally.

The United Kingdom (UK) had identified a variant called B.1.1.7 with a large number of mutations in late 2020. This variant spreads more easily and quickly than other variants.

In January 2021, experts in the UK reported that this variant may be associated with an increased risk of death compared to other variant viruses, but more studies are needed to confirm this finding. It has since been detected in many countries around the world. This variant was first detected in the US at the end of December 2020.

In South Africa, another variant called B.1.351 emerged independently of B.1.1.7. Originally detected in early October 2020, B.1.351 shares some mutations with B.1.1.7. Cases caused by this variant have been reported in the US at the end of January 2021.

In Brazil, a variant called P.1 emerged that was first identified in travellers from Brazil, who were tested during routine screening at an airport in Japan, in early January. This variant contains a set of additional mutations that may affect its ability to be recognized by antibodies. This variant was first detected in the US at the end of January 2021.

These variants seem to spread more easily and quickly than other variants, which may lead to more cases of COVID-19. An increase in the number of cases will put more strain on health care resources, lead to more hospitalizations, and potentially more deaths.

So far, studies suggest that antibodies generated through vaccination with currently authorized vaccines recognize these variants. This is being closely investigated and more studies are underway.

Rigorous and increased compliance with public health mitigation strategies, such as vaccination, physical distancing, use of masks, hand hygiene, and isolation and quarantine, is essential to limit the spread of the virus that causes COVID-19 and protect public health.

A total of 11,094 likely hospital-acquired covid-19 cases have been reported in the first 24 days of January, the latest data available. This is already higher than any other month in the second and third waves of covid.

The implications for UK Telemedicine November 2020 to 31 January 2021

Obviously, the fast roll-out of the vaccination programme has been heralded as a true saviour in the UK and the general public are getting excited about the possibility of life returning to normal with no face coverings and social distancing. Unfortunately, the reality is that COVID is here to stay for many years and the vaccinations are not 100% effective with efficacy between 50% and 95% being estimated. That means that people are still going to get infected, but in smaller numbers, and hospitals are still going to admit patients with COVID disease for treatment but hopefully they will be less ill than we have seen to date.

In addition we do have a problem with hospital acquired COVID infection and at 29th January 2021 it was known that 450 patients per day caught COVID in hospitals during January.

This means that a long-term plan to reduce contact and prevent cross-infection is still required because there will still be infected people in the community and there is concern that the new variants of COVID listed above (and others in the future) may become resistant to the vaccinated patients.

We believe that the recommendations for increasing the use of Telemedicine referred to in Chapter 14 are even more required in the future to reduce the number of people attending hospital and to reduce the possibility of cross-infecting patients who are visiting or admitted to hospital with COVID.

We would therefore recommend the following:-

A strategy should be developed for triaging patients at home via Telemedicine who might have COVID before considering transferring them to hospital. This might be done by using a combination of assessment parameters such as those developed by Prof Tim Spector's Covid Symptom Study app [3] and the use of a remote pulse oximeter in the patient's home.

A strategy to reduce General Practitioner and hospital out-patient visits by using Telemedicine consultations as an alternative but with properly designed Medical Telemedicine platforms – not just video-meeting room consultation which fail to provide appropriate patient documentation and document transfer facilities.

Journey of Telemedicine from being a Product to a Service and stepping into becoming a Telehealth Culture

Success of www.Doctors247.online as a successful Telemedicine remote healthcare delivery model, the Health Department of Punjab, the largest province with 110 million population formally approached Dr Suhail Chughtai to design a Telehealth Service Structure connecting Basic Health Unit in small towns and villages to the Specialist Doctors of District Headquarter Hospitals. The idea was to not only provide specialist care at the Basic Health Unit making life of the patient easy but also to off-load burden on District Hospitals OPD practice.

Dr Suhail Chughtai, designed a Telemedicine Service website, **www.SehatGhar.online** which was launched as a pilot in last quarter of 2020. Training of para-medical staff at the Basic Health Units and care-givers (Specialists) at the District Headquarter hospitals were trained in batches, both locally and by Dr Suhail Chughtai over e-class room. Till end of January, over 3000 patients have been treated by the Specialists through this website which has been deployed in Lahore Division of Punjab.

RADIO PAKISTAN   Tuesday, 30 June 2020, 9:48:03 pm   Search

HOME   NATIONAL   COVID-19   WORLD   BUSINESS   BUDGET 2020-21   SPORTS   CURRENT AFFAI

Sehat Ghar project to be started in seven districts of southern Punjab: Dr. Yasmin

June 27, 2020

Punjab Minister for Health, Dr. Yasmin Rashid has said that Sehat Ghar project will be started in seven districts of the southern Punjab.

She stated this while addressing a meeting in Lahore today (Saturday).

On this occasion, Special Secretary Ajmal Bhatti briefed her about functionality of Urban Primary Healthcare System and Sehat Ghar project.

The Minister said that Sehat Ghar will be functional after provision of facilities and the project will help provide better medical facilities to the masses.

She said that the Pilot Project of Tele Medicine will be run in Lahore.

She said that clinical audit is tremendously important which will improve the situation in public hospitals.

She said that recovery of patient is the key to success of doctors.

Dr Yasmin Rashid said that the patient ratio have been increased in public hospitals of province after better medication and health facilities there.

The plan is to take this onward to other 8 Divisions of the province of Punjab in the course of next few months. The Governor of Punjab recently launched the extension of the project in Sahiwal on 14th January 2020 at a ceremony hosted by the Principal Sahiwal Medical College, some four hours drive southwards from Lahore. The ceremony was participated by Dr Suhail Chughtai who visited Pakistan during that period.

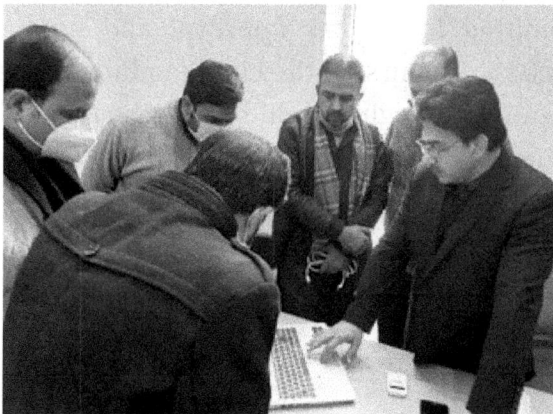

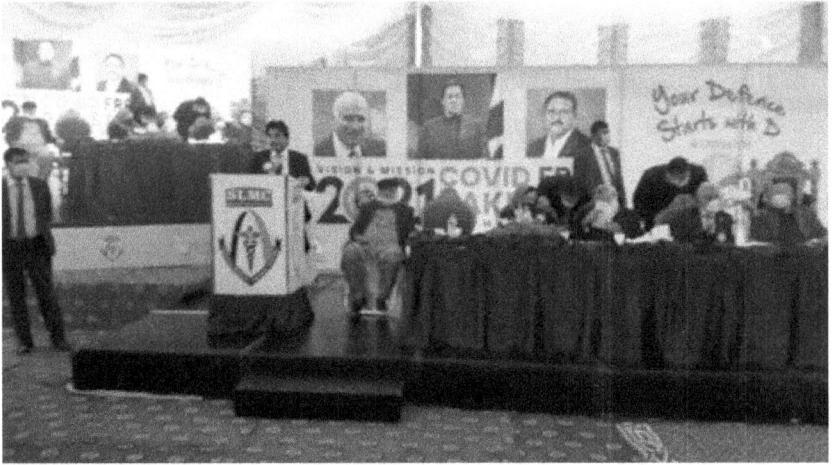

Setting up of Department of Health Informatics, Telehealth and Artificial Intelligence

The deliberations initiated back in March 2020 reached their completion in January 2021 at a visit to the University of Health Sciences, Lahore Pakistan by Dr Suhail Chughtai where the concept approval of the Department of Health Informatics, Telehealth and Artificial Intelligence was formally announced to Press and Media in a ceremony.

The design of the master's degree Course in the subject was submitted for higher approval and funding in late January 2021. The first of the eight modules of the master's degree Course to begin would be "Telehealth and e-Health Management", spanned over 64 hours of instructions lectures.

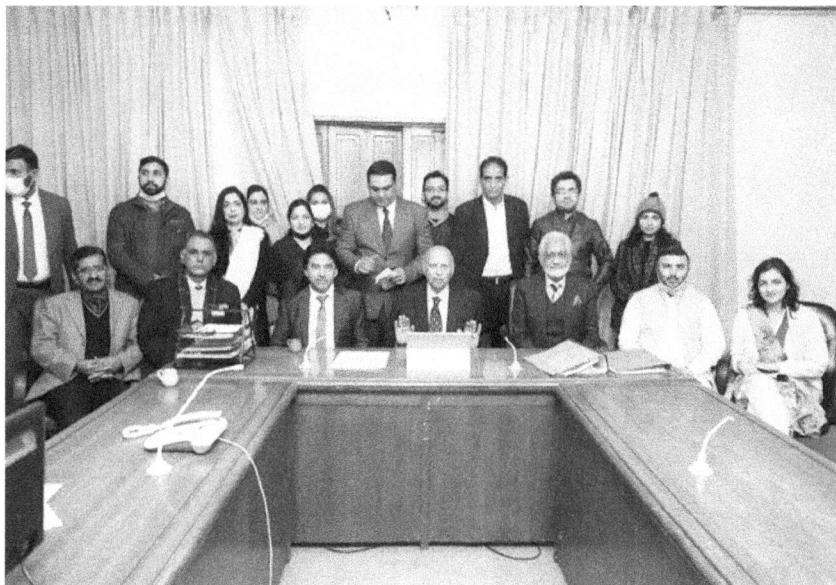

References

CDC, New Variants of the Virus that Causes COVID-19. 2021, Centers for Disease Control and Prevention, USA: CDC Website. https://www.cdc.gov/coronavirus/2019-ncov/transmission/variant.html

Discombe, M., Over 450 people a day caught covid in hospitals during January, in Health Service Journal, A. 2021, Health Service Journal (HSJ): https://www.hsj.co.uk/coronavirus/over-450-people-a-day-caught-covid-in-hospitals-during-january/7029404.article

Coombes, R. and T. Spector, The BMJ Interview: Tim Spector on how data can arm us against covid-19. British Medical Journal, 2020. 371(m4123): p. 1756-1833 www.bmj.com/content/371/bmj.m4123